A DENTAL PRACTITIONER HANDBOOK
SERIES EDITED BY DONALD D. DERRICK, D.D.S., L.D.S. R.C.S.

# ENDODONTICS IN CLINICAL PRACTICE

## F. J. HARTY
B.D.SC.(MELB.), L.D.S.(VICT.)

*Hon. Lecturer,*
*Department of Conservative Dentistry,*
*Institute of Dental Surgery,*
*University of London*

*with Chapters by*
### MALCOLM HARRIS
M.B., F.D.S. R.C.S.
### J. SAVILLE ZAMET
M. Phil., F.D.S. R.C.S.

BRISTOL : JOHN WRIGHT & SONS LTD.
1976

ISBN 0 7236 0439 8

PRINTED IN GREAT BRITAIN BY HENRY LING LTD., A SUBSIDIARY OF JOHN WRIGHT & SONS LTD., AT THE DORSET PRESS, DORCHESTER

ENDODONTICS IN CLINICAL PRACTICE

# PREFACE

FOR many years Endodontics has been the cinderella of dentistry and countless teeth have been extracted because an exposed or painful tooth was considered untreatable. The reasons why this attitude developed, and why it persists to the present day, are complex but the chief reason must be a lack of understanding of the basic principles of endodontic therapy.

The pulp represents the dentist's chief bugbear and, often, his orderly day is upset by a patient requiring emergency treatment because of a diseased pulp. A simple, quick but crude way of treating such a patient is by removing the pulp together with the tooth that surrounds it.

This is accepted as correct treatment by most patients and, alas, by a lamentably large section of the profession. Before patients can be influenced it is necessary for a section of the profession to change its attitude to endodontics. Far too many consider that success in Endodontics can only be achieved by sorcery and/or the use of the many magical and expensive potions and drugs readily available.

This book has been written for the general practitioner who is still frightened of the dental pulp and who blanches at the sight of a pulp exposure. Today's practitioner is yesterday's student and it is a matter of some regret that the general practitioner's attitude is the direct result of his undergraduate teaching. A pulp exposure was (and unfortunately, in some establishments, still is) considered a heinous crime and the student was made to feel that he could do no greater wrong. Very seldom was he taught how to save the tooth let alone the pulp.

I hope it will be clear to those who read this book that Endodontics is only an extension of conservative dentistry and that it should be practised by general practitioners and not by super specialists.

Much of the contents of this book owes its origin to notes prepared for the postgraduate students at the Institute of Dental Surgery and the Eastman Dental Hospital and I am most grateful to Professor G. A. Morrant for allowing me to use this material and also for his help and encouragement in the preparation of the text.

Dr. Malcolm Harris and Mr. John Saville Zamet have each contributed a chapter that bridges the gap between Endodontics and their specialized fields and I am indebted to both these gentlemen for their valuable contribution.

Mr. Alan Kinghorn and Mr. L. J. Leggett deserve special mention because the contents of this book is based on their teaching. Mr. Leggett has also read and corrected several of the chapters. Likewise I am indebted to Mr. T. R. Hill for his help with Chapter 8 and for allowing me to use *Figs.* 66, 67, 68.

I am grateful to Mr. D. H. Roberts and Professor J. H. Sowray for giving me permission to quote freely from their book '*Local Analgesia in Dentistry*'.

Many colleagues provided me with facts, opinions and information, and whilst it is not possible to name each one individually I would like to express my particular thanks to the following: Mr. J. E. Catling, Mr. M. R. Dimashkieh, Mr. D. B. A. Little, Mr. J. J. Messing, Mr. D. C. Rule, Mr. J. D. Strahan, Mr. W. M. Tay, Mr. R. Valentine, Mr. M. D. Wise and also to Mr. A. S. Atkinson, of the British Standards Institution, and to Mr. J. A. Donaldson, in his capacity as Honorary Curator of the museum of the British Dental Association, and for allowing me to photograph the instruments in *Fig.* 1.

It is said that the success of any book depends, to a large degree, on the quality of the illustrations. If this book is successful it will be due to the care taken by Mrs. Angela Christie in preparing the many line drawings and to Mr. J. W. Morgan and the staff of the Photographic Department of the Institute of Dental Surgery for the photography. I am also thankful to our Librarian Mrs. M. A. Cowperthwaite for checking the references.

It is appropriate that I pay a special tribute to Mrs. S. Morgan who assisted me greatly in the preparation and reading of the final typescript and also to Miss M. Cork, Miss V. Gwynne and to Mrs. J. Garrock-Jones for typing the many early drafts.

I am grateful to Mr. Donald Derrick for inviting me to contribute to the Dental Practitioner Series and to Mr. A. N. Boyd of John Wright & Sons Ltd. for his patience in awaiting delivery of the completed manuscript.

Finally, I must thank my wife and children for bearing with me so patiently and, in the case of Bryan, Warwick and Juliet, so very quietly whilst I was incommunicado in my study for endless weekends.

*July, 1975*                                                                                           *F.J.H.*

# CONTENTS

# CONTENTS

CHAPTER 1

# INTRODUCTION, HISTORY AND SCOPE OF THE SUBJECT

## INTRODUCTION

ENDODONTIC treatment can be defined as the treatment or the precautions taken to maintain the vital tooth, the moribund tooth or the non-vital tooth *in function* in the dental arch. This concept of treating the pulp of the tooth in order to preserve the tooth itself is a relatively modern development in the history of dentistry and it may be useful to review, very briefly, the history of pulp treatment in order to better appreciate modern thought on endodontic treatment.

Toothache has been a scourge to mankind from the earliest times. Both the Chinese and the Egyptians left records describing caries and alveolar abscesses. The Chinese considered that these abscesses were caused by a white worm with a black head that lived within the tooth. The 'worm theory' was current until the middle of the eighteenth century when Pierre Fauchard began to have doubts, but he could not express them forcibly because the Dean of the Medical Faculty, Antry, still believed the worm theory (Curson, 1965).

The Chinese treatment for an abscessed tooth was aimed at killing the worm with a preparation that contained arsenic. The use of this drug was taught in most dental schools as recently as the 1950s in spite of the realization that it was not self-limiting and that extensive tissue destruction occurred if minute amounts of the drug leaked into the soft tissues.

Pulpal treatment during Greek and Roman times was again aimed at destroying the pulp by cauterization, either with a hot needle, with boiling oil or with fomentation of opium and hyoscyamus.

The Syrian, Alchigenes, who lived in Rome about the end of the first century, realized that pain could be relieved by drilling into the pulp chamber in order to obtain drainage and he designed a trephine for this purpose. In spite of our modern 'wonder drugs' there is still no better method of relieving the pain of an abscessed tooth than the method advocated by Alchigenes.

Endodontic knowledge remained static until the sixteenth century when Vesalius, Fallopius and Eustachius described pulpal anatomy whilst still subscribing to the 'worm theory'.

1

In 1602, Jan van Haurne (Heurnius) and Pieter van Foreest, both practising in Leyden, appeared to differ in their views. The former still destroyed pulps with sulphuric acid whilst the latter was the first to speak of root canal therapy, and he suggested that the tooth be trephined and the pulp chamber filled with theriak (Prinz, 1945).

Thus until the latter part of the nineteenth century root therapy consisted of alleviating pulpal pain and the main function of the root canal was to provide retention for a pivot or dowel crown. At the same time bridgework became popular and many dental schools taught that no tooth should be used as an abutment unless it was first devitalized (Prinz, 1945). Root therapy became commonplace partly for the above reasons and also because the discovery of cocaine led to painless pulp extirpation. The method of cocaine pressure or contact pulpal anaesthesia appears to have originated with E. C. Briggs of Boston and described, more or less at the same time, by W. J. Morton, Ottolengui, Walkhoff, Buckley and others.

The injection of 4 per cent cocaine as a mandibular nerve block is attributed to William Halstead in 1884 (Roberts and Sowray, 1970).

The discovery of X-rays by Roentgen in 1895 and the first radiograph of the teeth by W. Koenig, of Frankfurt, in 1896, further popularized root therapy and gave the treatment a pseudo-scientific respectability.

About the same time dental manufacturers began to produce special root therapy instruments (*Fig.* 1) which were of the barb-broach variety and were used to remove pulp tissue or clean the canal of debris. As yet there was no concept of root filling the tooth and, as mentioned above, the object of the operation was to provide retention for a post crown of which the Richmond crown, the Davis crown and the Peeso split pin and tube were popular examples.

By 1910 'root therapy' had reached its zenith and no self-respecting dentist would extract a tooth. Every stump was retained and a porcelain or gold crown constructed. Fistulas appeared often and were treated by various methods for years on end if necessary. The connection between the fistula and the dead tooth was known but not acted upon.

In 1911 William Hunter attacked 'American Dentistry' and blamed bridgework for several diseases of unknown aetiology. He obtained several recoveries from these conditions by extracting the teeth of the patient. It is interesting to note that he did not condemn root therapy itself but rather the ill fitting bridgework and the sepsis that surrounded it.

About this time bacteriology became established and the findings of bacteriologists added fuel to the fire of Hunter's condemnations.

Radiography, which at first helped the dentist, now gave him irrefutable evidence of bony disease surrounding the roots of dead teeth.

Whilst the theory of focal infection was not enunciated by Billings until 1918, Hunter's condemnations started a reaction to root canal therapy and the wholesale removal of both non-vital and perfectly

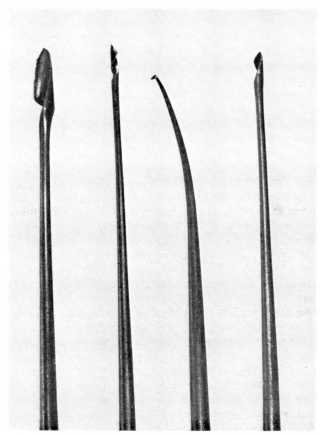

*Fig.* 1. Dr. Corydon Palmer's nerve instruments, which were designed to remove pulp tissue and prepare the canal for a post-retained restoration. (*Photograph by courtesy of Mr. J. A. Donaldson.*)

healthy teeth began. The blame for obscure diseases was placed on the dentition, and as dentists could not refute this theory they mutilated countless mouths. Naturally not all dentists accepted this wholesale dental destruction. Some, particularly on the continent of Europe, continued to save teeth in spite of the focal sepsis theory. It is difficult to know why Continental dentists disregarded this theory

3

and one explanation may be that Continental patients equated the loss of teeth with a loss of virility and therefore did not allow their dentists to mutilate their dentition. Alternatively it could be that Continental dentists were not as readily swayed by fashion as were their Anglo-Saxon colleagues.

## MODERN ENDODONTICS

The re-emergence of endodontics as a respectable branch of dental science began with the work of Okell and Elliott in 1935 and of Fish and MacLean in 1936. The former showed that the occurrence and degree of bacteriaemia depended on the severity of periodontal disease and the amount of tissue damage at operation. The latter showed the incongruity between bacteriological findings in the treatment of chronic oral infection and the histological picture. They showed that if the periodontal sulcus was cauterized before an extraction organisms could not be demonstrated in the bloodstream immediately postoperatively.

Gradually, the concept that a 'dead' tooth, i.e. a tooth without a pulp, was not necessarily infected began to be accepted. Further, it was realized that the function and usefulness of the tooth depended on the integrity of the periodontal tissues and not on the vitality of the pulp (Marshall, 1928).

Another important advance was made by Rickert and Dixon (1931) in their classic experiments which led to the formulation of the 'hollow tube' theory. They showed that an inflammatory reaction persisted around the hollow ends of steel and platinum hypodermic needles implanted in the skins of rabbits. Implanted solid materials, provided they themselves were not irritating either mechanically or chemically, showed no inflammatory tissue changes.

This realization that 'apical seal' was important led to the search for a filling material that was stable, non-irritant and provided a perfect seal to the apical foramen. Grove, in 1930, designed instruments that prepared a canal to a certain size and taper and used matching gold points to obturate the canal. Rickert and Dixon (1931), as an extension of their hollow tube investigations, formulated a sealer that contained an electrolytically precipitated silver.

Since then Jasper (1933), Green (1955a and b, 1956), Green (1957) and Ingle and Le Vine (1958) have attempted to formulate root filling points that would give the perfect apical seal. Unfortunately this ideal has not been achieved to date (Harty and Sandoozi, 1972).

Other important contributions to the rationale of endodontic therapy are a fuller knowledge of pulpal anatomy, (*see* Chapter 3), an appreciation of the importance of a sterile technique and the ease with which the root filling could be checked radiographically. These factors will be discussed fully in later chapters.

4

Until relatively recently endodontists were preoccupied with the effects of various potent drugs on the micro-organisms within the root canal and this preoccupation has diverted attention from the more pertinent endodontic problem, i.e. the effect of such drugs on the peridental tissues. All drugs that kill bacteria are also toxic to living tissue (Seltzer, 1971) and it is to be hoped that practitioners will realize this and abandon the use of harmful drugs for irrigation and medication of the root canal.

## SCOPE OF ENDODONTICS

The extent of the subject has altered considerably in the last 25 years. Formerly endodontic treatment confined itself to root filling techniques by conventional methods, and even apicectomy, which is an extention of these methods, was considered to be in the field of oral surgery.

Modern endodontics has a much wider field and includes the following:

1. The protection of the healthy pulp from disease or from chemical and mechanical injury.
2. Pulp capping (both direct and indirect).
3. Partial pulpectomy (pulpotomy).
4. Mummification.
5. Total pulpectomy (vital pulp extirpation).
6. Conservative root canal therapy of infected root canals.
7. Surgical endodontics which includes apicectomy, hemisection, root amputation, re-implantation of avulsed or subluxed teeth, elective replantation and endosseous endodontic implants.

REFERENCES

Billings F. (1918) *Focal Infection*. New York, Appleton.
Bremner M. D. K. (1954) *The Story of Dentistry*, rev. 3rd ed. New York, Dental Items of Interest Publishing.
Curson I. (1965) History and endodontics. *Dent. Pract. Dent. Rec.* **15**, 435.
Fish E. W. and MacLean I. (1936) The distribution of oral streptococci in the tissues. *Br. Dent. J.* **61**, 336.
Green D. (1955a) Morphology of the pulp cavity of permanent teeth. *Oral Surg.* **8**, 743.
Green D. (1955b) A stereo binocular microscopic study of the root apices and surrounding areas of 100 mandibular molars. *Oral Surg.* **8**, 1298.
Green D. (1956) A stereomicroscopic study of the root apices of 400 maxillary and mandibular anterior teeth. *Oral Surg.* **9**, 1224.
Green E. N. (1957) Microscopic investigation of root canal file and reamer widths. *Oral Surg.* **10**, 532.
Grove C. J. (1930) A simple and accurate procedure for the treating and filling of root canals. *J. Am. Dent. Assoc.* **17**, 1634.

Harty F. J. and Sandoozi A. E. (1972) The status of standardised endodontic instruments. *J. Br. Endodont. Soc.* **6**, 57.

Hunter W. (1911) The role of sepsis and antisepsis in medicine. *Lancet* **1**, 79.

Ingle J. I. and Le Vine M. (1958) The need for uniformity of endodontic instruments, equipment and filling materials. In: Grossman L. I. (ed.), *Transactions of the Second International Conference on Endodontics.* Philadelphia, University of Pennsylvania, p. 123.

Jasper E. A. (1933) Root-canal therapy in modern dentistry. *Dent. Cosmos* **75**, 823.

Marshall J. A. (1928) The relation to pulp-canal therapy of certain anatomical characteristics of dentin and cementum. *Dent. Cosmos* **70**, 253.

Okell C. C. and Elliott S. D. (1935) Bacteriaemia and oral sepsis with special reference to the aetiology of subacute endocarditis. *Lancet* **5**, 869.

Prinz H. (1945) *Dental Chronology: A Record of the More Important Historic Events in the Evolution of Dentistry.* London, Kimpton.

Rickert U. G. and Dixon C. M. (1931) The controlling of root surgery. In: *Transactions of the Eighth International Dental Congress, Paris.* Section IIIa, p. 15.

Roberts D. H. and Sowray J. H. (1970) *Local Analgesia in Dentistry.* Bristol, Wright.

Seltzer S. (1971) *Endodontology: Biologic Considerations in Endodontic Procedures.* New York, McGraw-Hill, p. 391.

# CHAPTER 2

# THE GENERAL AND SYSTEMIC ASPECTS OF ENDODONTICS

by Malcolm Harris, M.B., F.D.S. R.C.S.

*Consultant Oral Surgeon, King's College Hospital and Dental School, London*

## DENTAL PAIN: DIAGNOSIS, PREVENTION AND TREATMENT

A DETAILED case history is the most important aid to the diagnosis of any pain. Its aim should be to identify the affected tooth, estimate the degree of damage to its coronal insulation, the viability of the pulp, and the presence or absence of periodontal inflammation.

The principal pain characteristics to be established are:

1. *The quality:* Sharp pains of short duration suggest stimulation of exposed dentinal tubules. When such a pain recurs in the absence of any detectable coronal lesion one should suspect and seek a latent cusp fracture. These usually involve heavily filled upper premolars and lower first molars.

A dull continuous pain, either spontaneous or continuing after a provoking stimulus, implies hyperaemia of the pulp, and once this takes on a throbbing pulsatile character the pulp can be assumed to be acutely inflamed and irreversibly damaged. Necrosis of the neural elements or a spontaneous escape of the exudate may lead to a paradoxical cessation of all pain, which is often followed by facial swelling.

2. *Site and radiation:* It is important to remember that occasionally the referred pain or associated muscle spasm may be more prominent than pain in the tooth itself.

3. *Timing:* The total duration of the pain from its onset, the daily and nocturnal frequency and the length of each attack help to differentiate toothache from other types of pain. For instance, the temporomandibular joint dysfunction syndrome tends to give rise to intermittent attacks of prolonged pain, whereas trigeminal neuralgia, although an excruciating pain, is a series of very sudden paroxysms. Unlike toothache, both these conditions rarely disturb the patient at night.

4. *Provoking and relieving factors:* Sweet, sour, cold and hot food or drink classically provoke pulpal pain. Pain on walking or lying down suggests acute pulpal inflammation, whereas pain on biting and chewing points to periodontal inflammation.

5. *Associated features:* A swelling or a discharging sinus may help to localize the site of the trouble. The presence of food impaction between teeth will assist in distinguishing between a periodontal and a pulpal aetiology.

A careful examination must include the investigation of all tooth surfaces with a probe followed by occlusal and lateral percussion. Electric pulp testing and periapical radiographs are valuable secondary aids. The use of long cone techniques in the maxillary molar and premolar segments will help to eliminate superimposition and distortion of the root images. Suspicious multi-rooted teeth such as a maxillary first premolar should always be X-rayed from at least two angles in order to visualize both root apices (*see* Chapter 11). Not infrequently one encounters problems such as the partial death of a multi-canalled tooth giving rise to a diffuse or referred pain which is difficult to localize. Careful percussion followed by serial diagnostic injections of local anaesthetic can often help in such cases. Inject 1·5 ml over the apex of the suspected maxillary tooth. If the pain persists or is localized in the first instance to the lower quadrant, proceed with an infiltration at the mental foramen, followed if necessary after an interval of five minutes by an inferior dental block. Repeat your percussion of the teeth in both quadrants between each injection. In this way the source of pain can be traced to a maximum of three adjacent teeth. Furthermore, the patient's perception of the source of pain is invariably enhanced by this technique.

*Sinusitis*

Pain in a healthy tooth does occur but is uncommon and usually short-lived, unless the apex is adjacent to an inflamed antrum. A typical acute sinusitis is readily diagnosed when the toothache is associated with an upper respiratory tract infection, nasal obstruction and a post nasal discharge. However, with an isolated mono-sinusitis, tenderness over the antrum will be the only indication why apparently normal premolar or molar teeth are painful, tender to percussion and hypersensitive to pulp testing. Occasionally an additional feature is herpes labialis, suggesting that the 'quiet and isolated' sinus infection may be purely viral. An opaque antrum (*Fig.* 2) may be seen on an occipito-mental radiograph and will be the only means of confirming the diagnosis. Relief is best achieved with analgesics, inhalations of tinc. benz. co. or Karvol capsules repeated three times a day. An antibiotic such as tetracycline or ampicillin for 5 days will prevent an empyema.

Both the conventional and latent sinusitis are acute problems. Chronic sinusitis does not give rise to facial pain or swelling, nor mimic pulpal pathology.

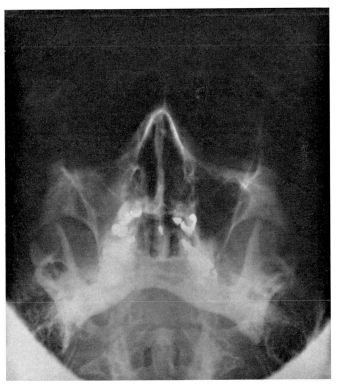

*Fig.* 2. An occipito-mental radiograph showing an opaque right antrum due to a non-exudative sinusitis.

*Idiopathic Periodontalgia*

In this condition (Harris, 1974) the patient may present with several tender teeth and more than one quadrant may be involved. The painful teeth ache or throb continuously and are readily provoked by thermal and mechanical stimuli. Relief with simple analgesics is variable but usually poor. Although the clinical history suggests pulpal pathology, examination and periapical radiographs invariably reveal no lesion. Furthermore extirpation of such a pulp offers no relief and even appears to aggravate the pain and so exploratory extirpations must be avoided. The pain may even persist after extraction of the tooth.

9

The pain mechanism is probably vascular in origin as some patients suffer from migraine, facial migrainous neuralgia or Raynaud's syndrome.

A psychogenic aetiology such as depression or rarely hysteria can often be established but in some cases this is not obvious. However, in all cases the pain is real and often severe.

Treatment should consist of reassurance, sedation or an anti-depressant drug, and analgesia with the avoidance of any dental procedures. Where bruxism is a contributory factor disengagement of the tender teeth with a Hawley bite guard (*Fig.* 3) may be of value.

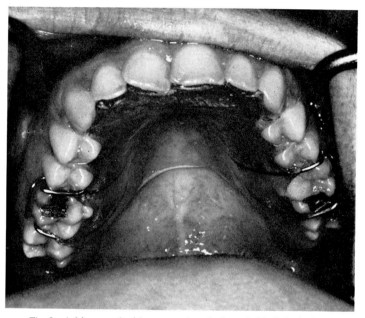

*Fig.* 3. A bite guard with an anterior platform behind the incisors to disengage the molar and premolar teeth on closure.

It is extremely important that an underlying emotional disorder should be considered and receive appropriate treatment before unnecessary and irreversible dental procedures are carried out.

*Pain Control during Operative Procedures*
Apprehensive individuals with tender inflamed tissues can be a problem. Where oral sedation and local analgesia have a limited effect the management of such a case is simplified by using intra-venous drugs. Analgesics such as pentazocine (Fortral) 30 mg or pethidine 50 mg can be administered by slow intravenous injection,

followed by 10–20 mg of diazepam (Valium) titrating the latter drug slowly until obvious sedation is achieved. This analgesic sedation reinforces the local analgesic which can then be given without distressing the patient.

*Pain Control after Endodontic Procedures and Apicectomy*
Most simple analgesics inhibit the release of inflammatory hormones such as the prostaglandins from damaged tissue which enhance both pain and oedema (Ferreira, 1972). These analgesics, in descending order of potency to counteract prostaglandin release, are: indomethacin, mefenamic acid, phenyl butazone and aspirin. Paracetamol has little anti-inflammatory effect.

Analgesics tend to work more effectively in a preventive role and help to maintain pain tolerance which falls with persistent pain. Therefore where appropriate a regular basic régime of postoperative pain control, such as mefenamic acid (Ponstan) 500 mg t.d.s. or two aspirin with codeine tablets for 2–5 days, should be employed. Any marked postoperative pain reaction usually means an inadequate and infrequent analgesic régime, and before resorting to potent narcotic analgesics the surgeon should establish that the patient is taking his medication as directed 4-hourly and supplement each dose of the simple analgesic with mild sedation such as diazepam (Valium) 2–5 mg. A regular combination of simple oral analgesics and sedation is invariably effective and well tolerated. This, of course, assumes that additional factors such as wound infection have been controlled and pus has been drained.

## ANGIONEUROTIC OEDEMA

Marked facial swelling in patients following root canal instrumentation is not uncommon even when covered by antibiotics. This reaction is strongly suggestive of an angioneurotic oedema and usually presents as a soft, relatively non-tender bloated lip or cheek. The sensitizing agent is probably necrotic pulpal products and such a swelling responds well to antihistamines such as chlorpheniramine maleate (Piriton) 4 mg t.d.s. and an appropriate antibiotic if one is not being used. A gross acute reaction should be given 10 mg chlorpheniramine intravenously or intramuscularly.

## INFECTION

*The Control of Infection*
As with pain the spread of infection is better prevented than cured. Penicillin and erythromycin remain the most useful antibiotics for orodental infections.

11

Approximately 1 per cent of the population is allergic to the 6-amino penicillinic acid nucleus which is present in *all* the penicillin analogues. Drugs taken by mouth and absorbed through the small intestine are less likely to give rise to severe allergic reactions than drugs given by injection, as the rise in blood level is slower and the

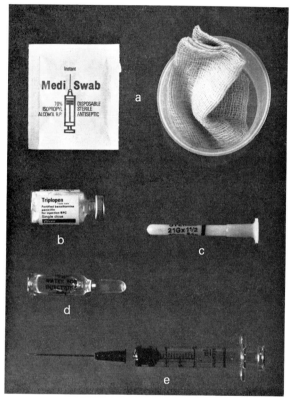

*Fig.* 4. The basic requirements for the administration of intramuscular antibiotics: *a*, Alcohol swabs; *b*, View of antibiotic; *c*, Intramuscular needle; *d*, Sterile water, 2 ml vial; *e*, Disposable 2 ml syringe.

peak lower. However, anaphylaxis is uncommon and the mortality rate has been reported as being as low as 1 : 65 000 (Idsoe et al., 1968). Therefore intramuscular antibiotics which ensure high blood levels in half an hour should be administered by the *dentist* where necessary. The basic requirements for intramuscular antibiotic therapy include (*Fig.* 4) (1) a selection of appropriate antibiotics, e.g. penicillin (1 mega unit of soluble) or a long acting preparation such as Triplopen.* Cephaloridine 0·5 g and lincomycin 0·6 g are useful alternatives for patients with a history of penicillin allergy. (2) 2 ml vials of sterile water for injection. (3) Disposable 2 ml syringes and intramuscular disposable needles.

The upper-outer quadrant of the buttock should be exposed and prepared with a swab soaked in surgical spirit, or isopropyl alcohol (*Fig.* 5). The needle should then be briskly and firmly 'stabbed'

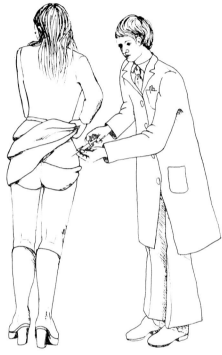

*Fig.* 5. Injection into the muscle mass of the upper outer quadrant of the buttock.

into the muscle mass. Always aspirate to exclude the possibility of entering a blood vessel prior to injection of the drug. The needle is then rapidly removed and the injection site rubbed firmly with the swab to seal the needle track.

The principal indications are prior to the drainage of pus from a grossly infected swelling or cyst or where a patient with a cardiac lesion (*see later*) requires a surgical procedure or the preparation of an infected root canal.

---

*Glaxo: benethamine penicillin G 475 mg.
      procaine penicillin 250 mg.
      sodium penicillin G 300 mg.

Loculated pus can be effectively aspirated with a broad bore intramuscular needle and disposable syringe. It avoids compression of the painful tissues and also enables the pus to be sent for bacteriological examination. Where pus is being aspirated from a cavity with rigid walls such as an intra-osseous cyst, a second needle should be inserted to act as an air vent. It is worth remembering that exudate from a mandibular tooth is often accessible by percutaneous aspiration. One should explore the facial swelling digitally in order to find an area of 'softening' or fluctuation through which the needle

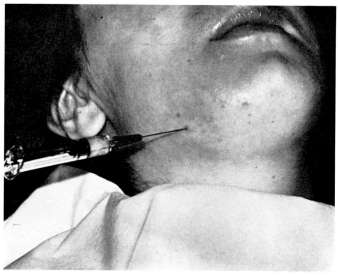

*Fig.* 6. Percutaneous aspiration of pus. Note the blanching of the area which has been previously anaesthetized with a small quantity of subcutaneous local anaesthetic.

is inserted. The drainage of pus by this method does not require a general anaesthetic and can be done with a small quantity of local analgesic injected submucosally for intra-oral or subcutaneously for extra-oral aspiration. Not only is the extra-oral technique pain free, but it does not leave a scar (*Fig.* 6). Apprehensive patients may require intravenous analgesia and sedation.

It is important to remember that sterile undrained pus following antibiotic therapy will continue to provoke pain and swelling.

Postoperative wounds and infected swellings need continued oral therapy such as phenoxymethyl penicillin 250 mg q.d.s. or erythromycin stearate* 250 mg q.d.s. or 500 mg b.d. for five days. An unresponsive cellulitis is usually indicative of undrained pus which

*Erythrocin 500: Abbott Laboratories.

must be evacuated and cultured to establish the need for a change of antibiotic. Antibacterial activity against *Staphylococcus aureus* such as flucloxacillin 250 mg q.d.s. may be required, but if the patient is allergic to penicillin one can use cephalexin 250–500 mg q.d.s. Allergy to the cephalosporins occurs in 8·2 per cent of patients allergic to penicillin but this is thought to be an independent sensitivity reaction rather than a cross reaction (Petz, 1971).

Another effective drug is clindamycin 150–300 mg q.d.s. which is a derivative of lincomycin and like lincomycin occasionally causes diarrhoea. Should this occur the drug must be replaced by an intramuscular antibiotic, and if severe the patient should be treated with tabs. diphenoxylate hydrochloride 2·5 mg with atropine sulphate 0·025 mg (Lomotil) t.d.s. and any necessary fluid replacement. The simplest régime for dehydration and electrolyte loss due to diarrhoea is a generous intake of orange juice.

Severe anaphylactoid reactions require 0·5–1 ml 1 : 1000 adrenaline to be given intramuscularly followed by hydrocortisone hemisuccinate 100 mg intravenously or intramuscularly. Mild reactions as discussed earlier (*see* p. 9) can be treated with antihistamines.

*Bacterial Endocarditis*

Concern about dental infection being the source of infective endocarditis has been expressed for many years (Horder, 1909). Fortunately despite widespread dental disease, bacterial endocarditis is uncommon, only one thousand cases occurring a year in England and Wales. Although the incidence of the disease has not altered appreciably the early mortality which was 100 per cent before the introduction of antibiotics is now 30 per cent (Hayward, 1973). The age range has also now extended and predisposing factors have increased from congenital, and rheumatic heart lesions to include arteriosclerotic valvular lesions and cardiac valve prostheses (Phillips and Eykyn, 1973).

Surprisingly enough, only 15 per cent have a detectable bacteriaemia of which only 44 per cent are due to *Streptococcus viridans*. Nonhaemolytic and micro-aerophilic streptococci and enterococci which may have originated in the mouth, gut, vagina or urinary tract have been cultured from the blood in the remainder. It is significant that 66 per cent of all cases appear to develop the disease without any precipitating cause, and furthermore edentulous cases are not infrequent (Croxson et al., 1971).

Hence the threat to the dental patient would appear to be small in the large population at risk and is probably determined by individual immunological competence rather than any particular dental procedure. Furthermore, endodontic procedures confined to the root canals do not produce a bacteriaemia (Bender et al., 1960).

## THERAPEUTIC GUIDE

ALLERGY    *Mild:*    chlorpheniramine
maleate (Piriton)    4 mg orally t.d.s.

      *Moderate:*    chlorpheniramine    10 mg intravenously or
maleate (Piriton)     intramuscularly
or hydrocortisone    100 mg intravenously or
hemisuccinate       intramuscularly
followed by prednisone 5 mg orally 4-hourly as
necessary

      *Severe:*    anaphylaxis. Adrenaline 0·5–1·0 ml of 1 : 1000
intramuscularly
followed by the steroid régime

PAIN    *Simple:*    soluble aspirin with
codeine       Tabs. 2, 4-hourly
mefenamic acid    2 capsules (500 mg)
(Ponstan)       4 hourly

      *Potent:*    pentazocine (Fortral)    50 mg orally 4-hourly
30 mg intramuscularly
or intravenously

      *Narcotic:*    pethidine    50 mg intramuscularly
or intravenously

SEDATION    diazepam (Valium)    2–5 mg orally 4-hourly
10–20 mg slowly
intravenously

INFECTION    *Oral:*    phenoxymethyl
penicillin       250 mg q.d.s.
erythromycin stearate    250 mg q.d.s.
or Erythrocin 500    500 mg b.d.
ampicillin       250 mg q.d.s.
flucloxacillin       250 mg q.d.s.
tetracycline       250 mg q.d.s.
clindamycin       150 mg q.d.s.
cephalexin       250 mg q.d.s.
For maximum effect oral antibiotics should be taken
6-hourly, e.g. at 06.00, 12.00, 18.00, 24.00 hours

      *Intramuscular:*    soluble penicillin G    1 mega unit
1 vial Triplopen (Glaxo)
cephaloridine       0·5 g
lincomycin       0·6 g

NASAL
DECONGESTANTS    tinc. benz. co.    4-hourly
Karvol (menthol)
capsules (Crookes)    4-hourly

DIARRHOEA    tabs. diphenoxylate
hydrochloride and
atropine sulphate
(Lomotil)       1, 4-hourly

But despite this margin of safety, endodontic and surgical procedures on susceptible patients such as those with valve lesions should be carried out under antibiotic cover and the completion of the tooth achieved in one session if possible. For absolute care, root canal therapy should be followed by an apicectomy to confirm the apical seal, and where this is deficient a retrograde seal should be inserted.

There is no evidence that the root filled tooth is any greater source of infection than the gingival sulcus.

For protection against a bacteriaemia a single injection of 600 000 U. of procaine penicillin intramuscularly one half hour prior to treatment or a vial of Triplopen (benethamine penicillin) is sufficient. Alternative antibiotics are cephaloridine 0·5 g or lincomycin 0·6 g i.m. The blood level achieved by phenoxymethyl penicillin 500 mg, erythromycin estolate 500 mg or clindamycin 300 mg taken orally one hour before treatment is also satisfactory in the absence of any gastro-intestinal upset. Some workers have suggested a broad spectrum antibiotic cover (Phillips and Eykyn, 1973) as the régime of choice, i.e. penicillin and streptomycin etc., but this has not been confirmed.

One short acting dose does not alter the oral flora significantly to produce resistant strains as does prolonged treatment and would therefore be appropriate for root canal therapy. However, the recommended alternative is to complete the treatment during a three day course of antibiotics to avoid the overgrowth of a resistant oral organism.

Patients receiving continuous penicillin therapy for the prevention of streptococcal sore throats which predispose to recurrent attacks of rheumatic fever will, of course, have a penicillin resistant oral flora and will require an alternative antibiotic.

An important exception to these procedures is a patient who gives a history of having had an episode of infective endocarditis. This would suggest a lack of immunological protection and should be considered a contra-indication to endodontic therapy.

*Immunosuppressive States*
Immunosuppressive drug therapy varies from the control of intractable asthma with small doses of corticosteroids to the maintenance of organ transplant recipients with several potent drugs.

Steroid therapy alone is no contra-indication to endodontic treatment except that it is important to control the extension of local infection with an antibiotic. There is also a theoretical possibility that an open root canal may become heavily contaminated with the yeasts which will require antifungal treatment. Corticosteroid supplements are required both during and twenty-four hours after any surgical procedure especially if pain and infection are prominent features. This may be done by doubling the drug dose for this period in consultation with the patient's physician.

Certain cases may be prone to septicaemia; these are patients on high doses of corticosteroids for severe collagen diseases such as disseminated lupus erythematosis, or in combination with cytotoxic drugs for malignant disease, or azathioprine for renal transplantation. As the risk of disseminating infection has not been evaluated under these conditions root canal therapy is contra-indicated and non-vital teeth should be extracted.

Radiotherapy for malignant disease of the jaws reduces both the vascularity and vitality of the alveolar bone. This is particularly evident in the mandible at sites receiving the maximum dose. Apart from the risk of non-vital infected teeth giving rise to an intractable osteoradionecrosis such teeth become extremely fragile and should be extracted prior to radiotherapy. Endodontic treatment to mandibular teeth after radiotherapy is similarly contra-indicated. It must be emphasized that all extractions after radiotherapy to the jaws should be done under antibiotic cover which is continued until the socket heals.

The maxillary teeth and alveolus do not usually receive the same maximum radiation dose except prior to maxillectomy. Therefore the greater vascularity and the smaller dose following therapy to the adjacent mandible should not exclude the possibility of careful endodontic therapy to maxillary teeth.


## CROSS INFECTION

Cross infection by non-disposable instruments remains a hazard in dentistry. Renewed interest has been stimulated by the introduction of tests capable of identifying serum hepatitis, hepatitis B, by means of its associated antigen, the so-called 'Australia antigen HBAg'.

This virus has been found to be carried predominantly by patients who are subjected to infusions of blood products or who have an impaired immunological mechanism.

Such patients include—

1. Patients in chronic renal failure requiring periodic dialysis.

2. Patients who have had organ transplants and who are maintained on immunosuppressive drugs.

3. Drug addicts.

4. Patients who give a history of having recently had Australia antigen positive hepatitis and are still positive when tested for the antigen.

Here the problem is twofold.
1. Contracting the virus oneself (Glenwright et al., 1974).
2. Communicating it with contaminated instruments to another patient (B.D.A., 1974).

The disease has a long incubation period of six weeks to six months and may finally present as a vague non-icteric illness. Nausea and abdominal discomfort precede the appearance of jaundice. The clinical course is variable but the condition usually lasts six weeks before the symptoms and signs begin to subside and the patient becomes antigen negative. Chronic liver disease and death, despite recent reports, are very rare and only a small percentage of patients remain Australia antigen positive suggesting a persistent carrier state (Williams, 1973). The danger probably arises mostly from those patients who are potent carriers, such as renal patients especially those on immunosuppressive drugs who can be shown to have a high HBAg titre. It would be unfair to deny these patients treatment especially as safe precautions are possible. A mask and rubber gloves should be worn and spectacles have also been recommended to protect viral entry through the conjunctiva by a contaminated aerosol. Although such a high infectivity of saliva has been questioned, the avoidance of inoculation of oneself or another patient with contaminated sharp instruments is important.

Where possible all instruments should be disposable, this is mandatory with needles and scalpel blades. Non-disposable instruments must be soaked in glutaraldehyde solution (Cidal), scrubbed and autoclaved at 120° C for 15 minutes or dry heat sterilized at 160° C for one hour. Boiling instruments is inadequate. This also means that only sterilizable hand pieces may be employed.


## MEDICO-LEGAL PROBLEMS

Endodontic instruments are small and the recumbent position of the patient together with digital fatigue can lead to their loss into the pharynx.

Aspiration is unlikely but has occurred. The alternative consequence of dropping a reamer into the stomach does not necessarily mean it will be passed harmlessly through the gut. To avoid unnecessary abdominal operations, rubber dam should always be used and is a better alternative to strings and chains attached to the reamer.

If such an accident does occur, immediate contact with a dental consultant can usually provide a convenient means to arrange for the retrieval of the instrument.

Failing this the Duty Surgical Officer at a local hospital should be contacted to order abdominal and chest radiographs and endoscopy.

Finally a detailed record of any misadventure should be made and a written report sent to your Defence Society.

REFERENCES

Bender I. B., Seltzer S. and Yermish M. (1960) The incidence of bacteremia in endodontic manipulation: Preliminary report. *Oral Surg.* **13,** 353.

British Dental Association. Dental Health Committee (1974) The prevention of transmission of serum hepatitis in dentistry. *Br. dent. J.* **137,** 28.

Croxson M. S., Altmann M. M. and O'Brien K. P. (1971) Dental status and recurrence of *Streptococcus viridans* endocarditis. *Lancet* **1,** 1205.

Ferreira S. H. (1972) Prostaglandins, aspirin-like drugs and analgesia. *Nature (New Biology)* **240,** 200.

Glenwright H. D., Edmonson H. D., Whitehead F. I. H. and Flewett T. H. (1974) Serum hepatitis in the dental surgeon. *Br. Dent. J.* **136,** 409.

Harris M. (1974) Psychogenic aspects of facial pain. *Br. Dent. J.* **136,** 199.

Hayward G. W. (1973) Infective endocarditis: A changing disease, I and II. *Br. Med. J.* **2,** 706 and 764.

Horder T. J. (1909) Infective endocarditis with an analysis of 150 cases and with special reference to the chronic form of the disease. *Q. J. Med.* **2,** 289.

Idsoe O., Guthe T., Willcox R. R. and De Weck A. L. (1968) Nature and extent of penicillin side reactions with particular reference to fatalities from anaphylactic shock. *Bull. WHO* **38,** 159.

Petz L. D. (1971) Immunologic reactions of humans to cephalosporins. *Postgrad. Med. J.* **47,** Suppl. 64.

Phillips I. and Eykyn S. (1973) In: Geddes A. M. and Williams J. D. W. (eds.), *Current Antibiotic Therapy: Bacterial Endocarditis following Cardiac Surgery.* Edinburgh, Churchill Livingstone, p. 113.

Williams R. (1973) Transmission of hepatitis and Australia antigenaemia within a liver unit. *Proc. R. Soc. Med.* **66,** 799.

CHAPTER 3

# PULP ANATOMY AND ACCESS CAVITIES

IN order to root fill a tooth successfully, it is essential to have a knowledge of the anatomy of the pulp cavity and of how this cavity can best be instrumented.

The study of pulp anatomy from radiographs alone is insufficient because radiographs show the form of the pulp cavity in two planes only, whereas a third plane exists in a labiolingual or buccolingual direction. Thus to appreciate fully the size, shape and form of pulp cavities it is necessary to study teeth in longitudinal sections mesiodistally and labio- or buccolingually. Transverse sections through the root at various levels are also essential if one is to know the shape of the root canal.

## NOMENCLATURE

Dissection of a tooth shows a central cavity, *the pulp cavity*, which resembles closely the outline of the tooth. As the cross-section of teeth is usually greater at the crown and tapers towards the apex, the pulp cavity follows the same general dimensions. The pulp cavity is usually described in two parts; the *pulp chamber*, which is that portion within the crown and the *pulp or root canal* which lies within the confines of the root.

*The pulp chamber* is always a single cavity and varies in shape according to the outline of the crown. Thus if the crown has well developed cusps, the pulp chamber projects into well developed *pulp horns*. In anterior teeth with well marked developmental grooves there are three pulp horns directed towards the incisal edge. These pulp horns are well developed in young teeth and gradually disappear with age.

*The pulp or root canals* are continuous with the pulp chamber and, normally, have their greatest diameter at the pulp chamber level. Because roots taper towards their apex, the canals also have a tapering form which ends in a constricted opening at the root end— the *apical foramen*. Sometimes a root has more than one foramen because the pulp may branch at its apical end and pass out of the root canal through these *multiple foramina*. The apical foramen rarely opens at the exact anatomical apex of the tooth, but about half to one millimetre from it. Generally, each root has only a single pulp canal. However, if roots fuse during development it is possible

21

to have two or more canals within the same root. For example, the mesial root of the lower first molar almost invariably has two canals which may end in a common foramen.

Since roots tend to be broader labio- or buccolingually than they are mesiodistally pulp cavities follow the same proportions and are often oval in cross section. Roots tend to become round in the apical third and thus pulp canals follow this outline and become circular in cross section.

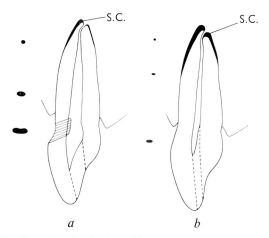

*Fig.* 7. Alteration of pulp size with age. *a*, Tooth of young adult. Note cross section of large pulp chamber with secondary dentine opposite carious lesion and relatively small deposits of apical secondary cementum (s.c.). *b*, Aged patient's tooth showing reduction in pulp size and further deposition of cementum thus altering the position of the apical foramen relative to the apex. Note also the cross sections of the root canals at various levels.

The *size* of the pulp cavity is influenced by the age of the patient and the amount of wear the tooth has experienced (*Fig.* 7). The *dental pulp* has the ability to react against injury by laying down 'secondary dentine' on the walls of the pulp chamber. This phenomenon occurs naturally as the patient grows older. Thus, children's teeth have the largest pulp cavities with well developed pulp horns. During the period of root development the root canal diameter is greater at the apex than at other levels of the root and is sometimes described as having a 'blunderbuss' appearance. As the tooth matures, the funnel-shaped foramen calcifies and constricts to a normal root shape with a small apical foramen.

Sometimes in old age or as a result of pathological changes the pulp cavity may be partially or entirely obliterated. Some authorities consider that calcification begins in the pulp chamber and proceeds apically and that even in extreme cases there still remains a fine residual canal in the apical half of the root. This may explain why a tooth with an apparently calcified canal may develop an apical radiolucent area.

## ACCESSORY AND LATERAL CANALS

These are formed during tooth development by the failure of dentine formation around blood vessels. *Accessory canals* are generally found in the apical third of the root and are branches of the main root canal. They end in accessory foramina and are more common in young patients because they become obliterated by cementum and dentine as the patient ages.

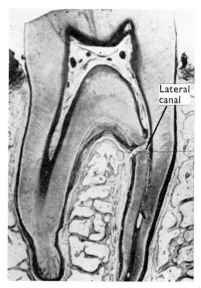

*Fig.* 8. Section of molar showing lateral canal close to furcation. (*From 'Orban's Oral Histology and Embryology'* 7th ed. *Courtesy of the Editor, Dr. H. Sicher, and C. V. Mosby Co.*, St. Louis.)

Accessory canals which open approximately at right angles to the main pulp cavity are termed *lateral canals* and are generally found in the furcation areas of posterior teeth (*Fig.* 8). The incidence of these canals is relatively high and Hess and Zurcher (1925) stated that their incidence was 17 per cent of all teeth. Lowman et al. (1973) report that patent lateral or accessory canals were present in the coronal or middle thirds of 59 per cent of molars. Kramer (1960), using a vascular injection technique, found that

23

lateral canals often had a greater diameter than the apical foramen and the blood vessels passing through lateral canals contributed more to the vascular system of the root canal than did the vessels entering through the apical foramen.

The presence of these canals has a bearing on the success rate of root therapy because it is not possible to instrument them through the main root canal and also because they are difficult to obturate with a root filling. Indeed, the only two methods by which such canals can be adequately sealed are either by a lateral condensation technique through the root canal or by a surgical approach when the accessory foramen is sealed directly from the outside of the root. Their importance in the periodontic/endodontic lesion is discussed fully in Chapter 10.

## THE APICAL THIRD OF THE ROOT (*Fig.* 9)

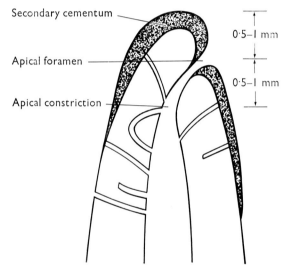

Secondary cementum

0·5–1 mm

Apical foramen

0·5–1 mm

Apical constriction

*Fig.* 9. Apical third of the root. Note that the apical foramen and the anatomical apex need not be coincident. The position of the apical foramen varies with age and can be 0·5–1 mm from the anatomical apex. Similarly the apical constriction can be 0·5–1 mm from the apical foramen.

Since the chief object of root therapy is to seal the canal contents from the periapical tissue, a knowledge of the anatomy of the apical third of the root is important.

It is a popular misconception that the apical foramen coincides with the anatomical apex of the tooth. This is an infrequent occurrence and usually the apical foramen opens half to one millimetre from the anatomical apex (Kuttler, 1955; Meyer, 1957; Chapman, 1969). This distance is not constant and may increase as the tooth ages because of the deposition of secondary cementum on the outer surface of the root and secondary dentine on the walls of the root canal.

The apical foramen is not always the most constricted portion of the root canal. Frequently the narrowest portion of the root canal, termed the *apical constriction*, occurs about half to one millimetre from the apical foramen (Chapman, 1969). Again the position of the apical constriction varies with age as deposits of secondary dentine, within the root canal, move the site of the constriction away from the apex. Ideally, the root filling should stop at this level and it is a good policy never to instrument, and thus destroy, this natural 'stop' to the root filling materials.

This alteration in the dimension and shape of the apical portion of the root canal with advancing age may be a factor in the increased success rate of conventional root therapy in older patients (Harty et al., 1970). Canals in such patients are easier to instrument to a circular cross section and as the canal and apical foramen are constricted it may be more difficult to instrument past the apical constriction and thus push infected material into the periapical tissues.

## PULP CAVITY ANATOMY AND ACCESS CAVITIES

The illustrations accompanying the descriptions of pulp cavity anatomy represent:

1. Longitudinal mesiodistal sections viewed from the lingual.

2. Longitudinal labio/buccolingual/palatal sections viewed from the mesial and, also, the axial angulation of the tooth relative to a horizontal occlusal plane.

3. Horizontal sections through the root(s)
   *a.* Three millimetres from apex
   *b.* At cervical level.

4. Incisal or occlusal view with outline of access cavity (dotted line).

1, 2 and 3 show dimensions and cross section of pulp cavity shortly after completion of root formation (shaded area) and in old age (black area).

## *Maxillary Central and Lateral Incisor (Figs.* 10, 11)

These are considered together because the outlines of these teeth and hence the pulp cavities, are similar. There are, of course, variations in size and central incisors are on average 23 mm long whilst laterals are about 22 mm. It is extremely rare for these teeth to have more than one root canal.

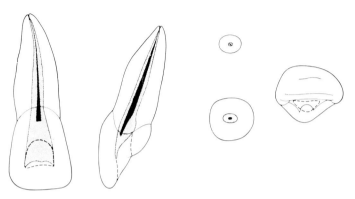

*Fig.* 10. Maxillary central incisor.

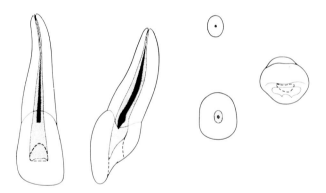

*Fig.* 11. Maxillary lateral incisor.

*The pulp chamber*, when viewed labiolingually, is seen to be pointed toward the incisal and widest at the cervical level. Mesiodistally both teeth follow the general outline of their crown and are thus widest at their incisal levels.

The central incisors of young patients normally show three pulp horns. Lateral incisors usually have two pulp horns and the incisal outline of the pulp chamber tends to be more rounded than that of central incisors.

*The root canal* differs greatly in outline when sectioned mesio-distally and buccolingually. The former section generally shows a fine straight canal and this is the view seen on X-ray (*Fig.* 12*a*). Buccolingually the canal is very much wider and often shows a constriction just below the cervical level. This view is never seen on X-rays and it is as well to remember that all canals have this third dimension which must be mechanically instrumented, cleansed and prepared to receive the final obturating root filling (*Fig.* 12*b*).

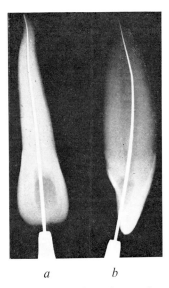

*a*       *b*

*Fig.* 12. *a*, Mesiodistal X-ray view of upper lateral incisor with diagnostic reamer showing a relatively straight canal. *b*, Bucco-lingual X-ray view of the same tooth showing wide cross section of canal. This view is not normally seen clinically. Note that the incorrect access cavity design results in the bending of the instrument which makes débridement of the lingual wall of the canal difficult if not impossible.

The canal is tapering in shape with an oval or irregular cross section cervically which gradually becomes round toward the apex.

There is generally very little apical curvature in central incisors and where it is present it is usually distal or labial. However, the apex of lateral incisors is often curved, generally in a distal direction.

As the tooth ages the anatomy of the pulp cavity alters with the deposition of secondary dentine. The roof of the pulp chamber recedes and may be at cervical margin level. The canal appears to be very narrow mesiodistally on X-ray. However, if one remembers

27

that the diameter labiolingually is much greater than in the mesio-distal plane one will appreciate that it is often possible to negotiate a canal which appears very fine or is apparently non-existent on the preoperative radiograph.

### Maxillary Canine (Fig. 13)

This is the longest tooth in the mouth and is, on average, 26·5 mm. It seldom has more than one root canal.

*The pulp chamber* is quite narrow and since there is but one pulp horn it is pointed incisally. The general shape of the pulp cavity is similar to the central and lateral incisors but as the root is much wider labiolingually the cavity follows this outline and is much wider in this plane than it is mesiodistally.

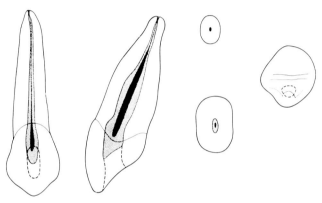

*Fig.* 13. Maxillary canine.

*The root canal* is oval and does not begin to become circular in cross section until the apical third. The apical constriction is not as well defined as in the central and lateral. This, together with the fact that often the root apex tapers and becomes very thin, makes canal length measurement difficult. The canal is usually straight but may show, apically, a distal curvature and less frequently a labial curvature.

### Access Cavities for the Maxillary Incisors and Canines

Access cavities in anterior teeth will vary in size and shape according to the dimension of the pulp. They should be designed so that root therapy instruments can reach to within 1 mm of the apical foramen without bending or binding against the walls of the access cavity or root canal. Débridement through a Class III cavity is rarely successful (*Fig.* 14) because the instrument binds against the access

28

cavity and may form a false canal apically which can lead to perforation. With this type of cavity it is usually not possible to include the pulp horn within the preparation and this site remains a source of infection to the remainder of the root canal.

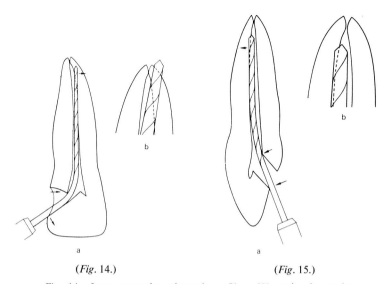

(*Fig.* 14.)          (*Fig.* 15.)

*Fig.* 14. Instrumentation through a Class III cavity is rarely successful because the instrument binds against the cavity walls and also because the tip of the instrument may form a step *a*, or even perforate the root *b*.

*Fig.* 15. *a*, The cingulum access cavity leads to apical step formation because of the excessive bending of the reamer or file. It also allows infected debris to remain hidden in the pulp chamber and pulp horns. *b*, Apical step formed on labial aspect of root canal.

Likewise an access cavity that is too close to the cingulum leads to sharp bends in the instrument with binding against the access cavity walls and possible step formation and/or perforation apically (*Fig.* 15). The commonly taught practice of gaining access to the pulp chamber through the cingulum is an anachronism from the days of the foot engine when, as well as being the shortest distance into the pulp chamber, it was also the only area where a slowly rotating bur could cut enamel without slipping off the tooth.

Ideally, the access cavity should extend far enough incisally to allow the unimpeded progress of the instrument to the apical area (*Fig.* 16). Sometimes the incisal edge has to be involved if access is to be adequate. No harm is done if the tooth is badly stained or carious thus requiring restoration with a post crown on completion of the root filling. Difficulties arise when the crown is sound and of good colour and a compromise has to be reached by limiting the incisal extension of the access cavity just short of the incisal edge. There are occasions where compromise is not possible and it is better to repair the damage to the incisal, and even to the labial surface, with a composite filling (or even with a crown) rather than jeopardize the root filling by inadequate access.

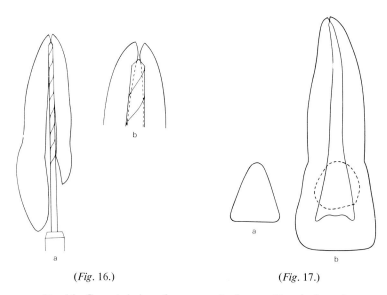

(*Fig.* 16.)                    (*Fig.* 17.)

*Fig.* 16. Correct design of access cavity for maxillary incisor. It extends far enough incisally to allow the unimpeded progress of the instrument to the apical area (*a*). Instrumentation should stop at the apical constriction (*b*).

*Fig.* 17. (*a*) Represents the correct access cavity outline viewed from the lingual aspect. If the design of the cavity is inadequate, as with the dotted line at (*b*), infected material will remain in the pulp chamber and may be transferred into the root canal during subsequent instrumentation.

As the pulp chamber is broader incisally than it is cervically the outline should be triangular and must extend far enough mesially and distally to include the pulp horns (*Fig.* 17).

Once adequate access has been made into the pulp chamber the cervical constriction should be removed by filing in order to make the instrumentation of the apical area easier.

Correct access cavity design is particularly important in the older patient because narrow root canals require the use of fine instruments which may break if bent excessively. Since the roof of the

30

pulp chamber is narrow and often at cervical level it is wise to begin the access cavity rather closer to the incisal edge than normally so that the pulp chamber can be approached in a straight line. This approach has the added advantage of minimum tooth destruction.

### *Maxillary First Premolar* (*Fig.* 18)

This tooth usually has two well developed fully formed roots which normally begin in the middle third of the root. It may also be single rooted. Irrespective of its outward form the tooth normally has two canals and in the case of the single-rooted specimen, these canals may open through a common apical foramen. In a small percentage of cases the tooth may be three rooted with three distinct canals, two buccally and one palatally.

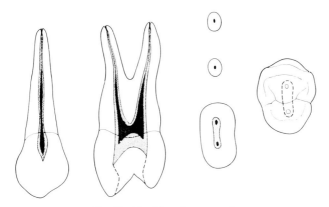

*Fig.* 18. Maxillary first premolar.

The average length of first premolars is 21 mm, that is just shorter than second premolars.

*The pulp chamber* is wide buccolingually with two distinct pulp horns. In mesiodistal section the pulp chamber is much narrower. The floor is rounded with the highest point in the centre and generally just below the level of the cervical margin. The orifices into the root canals are funnel-shaped and lie buccally and palatally.

*The root canals* are normally separate and very rarely blend into the ribbon-like type of canal frequently seen in the second premolar. They are usually straight with a round cross section.

As the tooth ages the dimensions of the pulp chamber do not alter appreciably except in a cervico-occlusal direction. Secondary dentine is deposited in the roof of the pulp chamber and this has the effect of bringing the roof very much closer to the floor. The floor level remains below the cervical area of the root and the thickened roof may now be below cervical level as well.

### Maxillary Second Premolar (*Fig.* 19)

This tooth normally has one root with a single canal. Very infrequently two roots may be present and whilst the outward appearance may be similar to the first premolar the floor of the pulp chamber extends well apically of the cervical level. The average length of the second bicuspid is slightly longer than the first and averages 21·5 mm.

The *pulp chamber* is wide buccopalatally and has two well defined pulp horns. Unlike the first premolar the floor of the pulp chamber extends apically well below the cervical level.

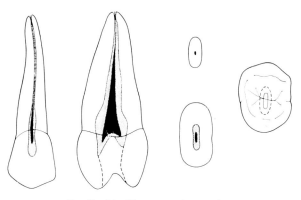

*Fig.* 19. Maxillary second premolar.

*The root canal* is wide buccopalatally and narrow mesiodistally. It tapers apically but rarely develops a circular cross section except for the apical two or three millimetres. Often the root canal of this single rooted tooth branches into two sections in the middle third of the root. These branches almost invariably join to form a common canal which has a relatively large foramen.

The canal is usually straight but the apex may curve to the distal and less frequently to the buccal.

As the tooth matures the roof of the pulp chamber recedes away from the crown and the remarks made for the first bicuspid apply equally to this tooth.

*Access Cavities for the Maxillary Premolars*

This should always be through the occlusal surface. Existing Class II or Class V cavities are unsatisfactory because saliva control is difficult and, in the case of the Class V, endodontic instruments have to be bent acutely in order to reach the apex of the tooth.

The shape of the access cavity is ovoid in a buccolingual direction. In the case of the first premolar the orifices of the root canal are readily visible as they lie just below the cervical margin level. The second premolar root canal is ribbon-shaped and, because it lies well below the cervical level, may not be readily visible.

Because the pulp horns in both teeth can be well developed it is easy when cutting a shallow occlusal cavity to expose the pulp horns and assume, wrongly, that these are the orifices of the root canal.

### *Maxillary First Molar* (*Fig.* 20)

The maxillary first molar normally has three root canals corresponding to the three roots. Of these, the palatal canal is the longest and is, on average, 21 mm.

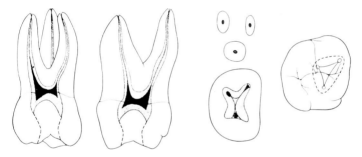

*Fig.* 20. Maxillary first molar.

*The pulp chamber* is quadrilateral in shape and wider buccopalatally than mesiodistally. It has four pulp horns, of which the mesiobuccal is the longest and sharpest in outline. The distobuccal pulp horn is smaller than the mesiobuccal but larger than the two palatal pulp horns.

The floor of the pulp chamber is normally just below the cervical level and is rounded and convex towards the occlusal. The orifices into the pulp canals are funnel-shaped and lie in the middle of the appropriate root.

Because the angle between the crown and the root varies in different teeth the relative position of the canal orifices will also vary. From *Fig.* 21 it will be seen that if the mesial and distal roots are near parallel to each other in the long axis of the tooth the orifices

33

into the canals are further apart, relative to each other, than they would be if the roots were widely divergent. Thus careful examination of the preoperative radiographs will give a clue to the position of the canal orifices.

Further it must be remembered that the cross section at cervical and mid-crown level are of different shape (i.e. the cervical shape is rhomboid rather than quadrilateral). For this reason the mesio-buccal canal opening is closer to the buccal wall than is the disto-buccal orifice. For the same reason the distobuccal root (and hence the opening into the root canal) is closer to the middle of the tooth than to the distal wall. The palatal root canal orifice lies in the middle of the palatal root and is normally easy to identify.

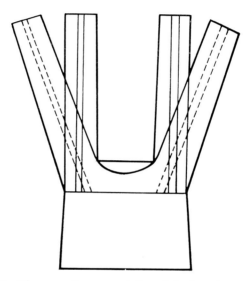

*Fig.* 21. Diagrammatic representation of the buccal roots of the maxillary molar. As roots diverge so orifices into root canals lie closer together.

The cross sections of the root canals vary considerably. The mesio-buccal canal is usually the most difficult to instrument because it leaves the pulp chamber in a mesial direction. It is elliptical in cross section and narrower in the mesiodistal plane. Instrumentation is further complicated because this canal can often split into two irregular branches which may join again before reaching the apical foramen. These branches lie in a buccopalatal plane and are thus superimposed on the preoperative X-ray, which makes diagnosis difficult. A further complication occurs because the mesiobuccal root often curves distopalatally in the apical third of the root.

The distobuccal canal is the shortest and finest of the three canals and leaves the pulp chamber in a distal direction. It is ovoid in shape and again narrower mesiodistally. It tapers towards the apex and becomes circular in cross section. The canal normally curves mesially in the apical half of the root.

The palatal canal is the largest and longest of the three canals and leaves the pulp chamber as a round canal which gradually tapers apically. In about 50 per cent of roots it is not straight but curves buccally in the apical 4 or 5 millimetres. This curvature is, of course, not apparent on X-ray.

As the tooth ages the canals become much finer and the orifices into the canals more difficult to find. Secondary dentine is deposited chiefly on the roof of the pulp chamber and to a lesser degree on the floor and walls. Thus the pulp chamber becomes very narrow between roof and floor. This fact may lead to problems during access cavity preparation for it is relatively easy (particularly with ultra high speed instrumentation) to perforate the roof of the chamber, and, because the distance between the floor and roof is so small, to continue cutting past the floor and into the periodontal ligament. To prevent this accident it may be wise to restrict the use of turbine instrumentation to enamel and to complete the access cavity with a round bur in a slowly rotating handpiece.

## Maxillary Second Molar (Fig. 22)

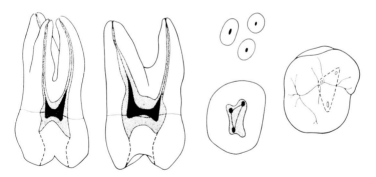

Fig. 22. Maxillary second molar.

The maxillary second molar is usually a smaller replica of the first molar, although the roots are more slender and proportionally longer—the palatal root being on average 20·5 mm. As the roots do not spread as widely as in the first molar, the root canals are generally less curved and the distobuccal canal orifice is usually found closer to the centre of the tooth. The roots of the tooth may be fused but irrespective of this the tooth normally has three root canals.

## Maxillary Third Molar

The morphology of this tooth differs considerably and can vary from a near replica of a second molar to a single rooted cuspid-like tooth. Even when the tooth is well formed, the number of root canals deviates considerably from the normal in other maxillary teeth. For these reasons, and also because access to upper wisdom teeth is difficult, it may not be suitable for conventional root canal therapy and, if it is imperative that the tooth be retained, a mummification technique may prove useful.

### Access Cavities to the Maxillary Molars

In designing access cavities for molar teeth, it is as well to remember that the object of root therapy is to maintain teeth *in function*. Thus the unnecessary destruction of coronal tooth substance inevitably leads to a weakening of the tooth which may fracture even if 'protected' by a cast metal restoration. Thus the cardinal rule in access cavity design is to remove the minimum amount of tooth substance required to visually identify the orifices of the root canals and also to allow unimpeded instrumentation of the apical areas of these canals. The pulp horns must also be removed to prevent infected material from remaining in these areas.

The access cavity outline for maxillary teeth is triangular with the base of the triangle towards the buccal and the apex palatally. Because the distobuccal canal is not as close to the buccal surface as the mesiobuccal canal, less tooth need be removed from this area.

The occlusal half of the access cavity should be similar in design to a Class I inlay cavity. The walls should not be undercut but should flare occlusally. This precaution will prevent the accidental forcing of the temporary filling into the pulp chamber during mastication and thus prevent medicaments from being forced periapically.

The canal openings generally lie within the mesial two-thirds of the crown and thus the access cavity need not be extended too far distally.

### Mandibular Central and Lateral Incisor (*Figs.* 23, 24)

These are considered together because the general outline and hence the pulp cavities are very similar. Both teeth are on average 21 mm long although the central is normally a little shorter than the lateral incisor. Usually there is only one straight uncomplicated canal

36

present. However, the lateral incisor particularly often divides in the mid-third of the root to give a labial and lingual branch. Because of their position these branches are not visible on X-ray and this second canal may be the cause of unexplained root canal therapy failure where it is missed during instrumentation.

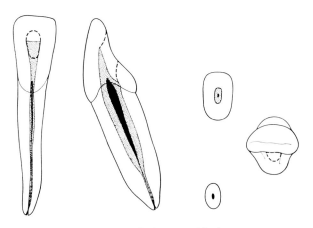

Fig. 23. Mandibular central incisor.

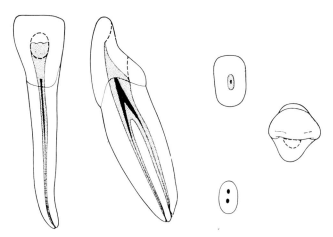

Fig. 24. Mandibular lateral incisor.

*The pulp chamber* is a smaller replica of the upper incisors. It is pointed incisally with three pulp horns which are not well developed and is oval in cross section and wider labiolingually than it is mesiodistally.

37

*The root canal* is normally straight but may curve to the distal and less often to the labial. It does not begin to constrict until the middle third of the root when it becomes circular in outline. The tooth ages similarly to the upper incisors and the incisal portion of the pulp chamber may recede to a level below the cervical margin.

## Mandibular Canine (*Fig.* 25)

Again this tooth, and hence the pulp cavity, resembles the maxillary canine although it is smaller in all dimensions. The average length is 22·5 mm.

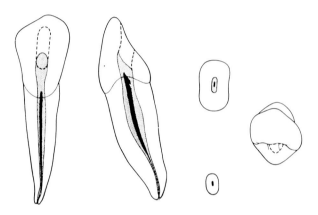

*Fig.* 25. Mandibular canine.

*The pulp chamber and root canal* are generally similar to the maxillary canine, the only difference being that the canal is more likely to be straight with rare distal apical curvatures. Very infrequently this root canal may divide into two branches in the same manner as the other lower incisors.

### Access Cavities to Mandibular Incisors and Canines

Essentially these are identical to the upper incisors. However, because of the more pronounced labial curvature of the crown of the central and lateral and also because the canals (particularly in the older patient) are so fine it is sometimes necessary to involve the incisal edge of the tooth so that instruments may reach the apical 2 or 3 mm without being bent.

## Mandibular Premolars (*Figs.* 26, 27)

These teeth are described together because, unlike the upper premolars, they are similar in outline and pulp cavity form.

Normally, there is a single root canal which in a small percentage of specimens may divide temporarily in the mid-third to form two branches which rejoin near the apical foramen.

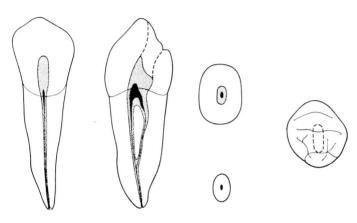

*Fig.* 26.  Mandibular first premolar.

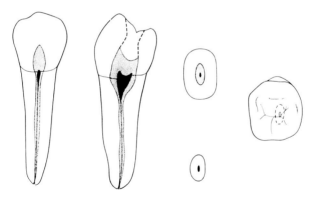

*Fig.* 27.  Mandibular second premolar.

*The pulp chamber* is wide buccolingually and whilst there are two pulp horns only the buccal is well developed.  The lingual pulp horn is very slight in the first premolar (because the lingual cusp is rudimentary) and better developed in the second premolar.

39

*The pulp canal.* The canals of these two teeth are similar, although smaller than the canines, and are thus wide buccolingually until they reach the middle third of the root, when they constrict to a circular cross section. As was mentioned before, the canal may temporarily branch in the middle third and rejoin near the apical foramen. The canal may be quite curved in the apical third of the root, usually in a distal direction.

### Access Cavities to Mandibular Premolars

This is essentially the same as for maxillary premolars and again must be through the occlusal surface.

### Mandibular First and Second Molar *(Figs. 28, 29)*

Since these two teeth resemble each other more than the corresponding upper teeth they will be described together.

Normally, both teeth have two roots, a mesial and a distal. The latter is smaller and rounder than the mesial. Both teeth usually have three canals. The first molar is an average 21 mm whilst the second is usually 1 millimetre shorter.

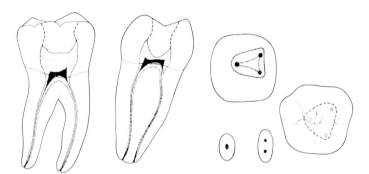

*Fig.* 28. Mandibular first molar.

*The pulp chamber* is wider mesially than it is distally and has five pulp horns in the case of the first molar and four in the second molar, the lingual pulp horns being longer and more pointed.

The floor is rounded and convex toward the occlusal and lies just below the cervical level. The root canals leave the pulp chamber through funnel-shaped openings of which the mesial are much finer than the distal.

*The root canals.* The mesial root has two canals, the mesiobuccal and the mesiolingual. It is said that the former canal is the most difficult canal to instrument and this is so because of its tortuous path. It leaves the pulp chamber in a mesial direction which alters to a distal direction in the middle third of the root. Frequently, as well as turning distally the canal also turns lingually. Unless these 'twists' in the root canal are appreciated and the reamer or file bent accordingly, 'step' formation may result which makes instrumentation past the 'step' difficult. Instrumentation is made more difficult by the fine circular cross section of the canal.

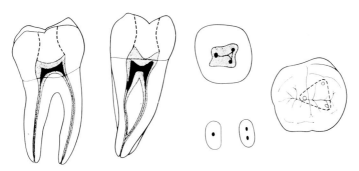

*Fig.* 29. Mandibular second molar.

The mesiolingual canal is slightly larger in cross section and generally follows a much straighter course although it may curve mesially in the apical area. These canals may join in the apical fifth of the root and end in a single foramen.

To check whether the mesial canals join or remain separate one places an instrument into one canal, just short of the apical foramen, and an attempt is made to instrument the other canal to its correct level. If the instrument binds short of this level one can safely assume that the canals join at that point and will lead to a common apical foramen.

The distal canal is usually larger and more oval in cross section than the mesial canals. It is generally straight and presents few problems of instrumentation. A small number of teeth have two distal canals lying in a buccal and lingual position. These twin canals are usually found in individuals with large well formed molars, which are often square in outline. If the first molar has twin distal canals, then it is likely that the second molar will do so as well.

As the tooth ages the canals become more constricted and, as with maxillary molars, the roof of the pulp chamber recedes from the occlusal surface.

41

## Mandibular Third Molar

This tooth is often malformed with numerous and/or poorly developed cusps. It generally has as many root canals as there are cusps. The root canals are generally larger than in other molars probably because the tooth develops later in life. The roots and thus the pulp canals are short and poorly developed.

In spite of the above shortcomings it is generally less difficult to root fill mandibular than maxillary wisdom teeth because access is easier due to the mesial inclination of these teeth and also because they are more likely to follow the normal anatomy of the second molar rather than an aberrant form.

### Access Cavities to Mandibular Molars

The basic principle is again the conservation of as much tooth as possible. Ideally the cavity should be triangular in shape with the base of the triangle towards the mesial. Care must be taken to remove the entire roof of the pulp chamber lest infected material be trapped beneath the remaining pulp horns. Nevertheless, the distally situated apex of the cavities need not extend much further than the central pit because of the distal angulation of the distal root canal (*Figs.* 28, 29) makes instrumentation relatively easy.

Sometimes it is suggested that the mesiobuccal cusp be removed completely to give better access to the mesiobuccal canal. Whilst this may improve visual identification of the root canal opening, it very seldom helps with actual instrumentation when one remembers that the initial direction of the root canal is mesial. Decuspation makes saliva control more difficult, whether it be by rubber dam or by other means, and thus it rarely serves a useful purpose.

As for other posterior teeth, the 'inlay' type access cavity prevents masticatory forces from dislodging a temporary filling towards the pulp.

# PULP CAVITY ANATOMY OF
# THE DECIDUOUS DENTITION

An intimate knowledge of the deciduous pulp cavity anatomy is not essential in order to carry out root therapy in primary teeth. Whilst the object of root therapy in both the permanent and deciduous dentition remains the same, i.e. the preservation of the tooth in function, the technique used to achieve this differs considerably. In the permanent dentition the aim is to seal the apical foramen with a non-resorbable material, whilst in the deciduous dentition care is taken to fill the root canal with a resorbable root filling, which will resorb at the same rate as the root.

42

The deciduous pulp cavities have certain common characteristics:

1. Proportionally they are much larger than in the permanent dentition.
2. The enamel and dentine surrounding the pulp cavities are much thinner than in the permanent dentition.
3. There is no clear demarcation between the pulp chamber and the root canals.
4. The pulp canals are more slender and tapering, and are longer in proportion to the crown, than the corresponding permanent teeth.
5. Multi-rooted deciduous teeth show a greater degree of interconnecting branches between pulp canals.
6. The pulp horns of the deciduous molars are more pointed than the cusp anatomy suggests.

### *The Deciduous Incisors and Canines (Fig. 30)*

The pulp chambers of both upper and lower incisors and canines follow closely their crown outlines. However, the pulp tissue is much closer to the surface of the tooth, and the pulp horns are not as sharp and pronounced as in the permanent dentition.

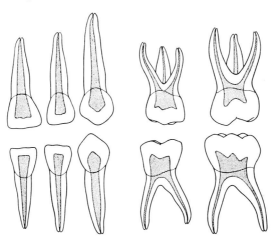

*Fig.* 30. Pulp anatomy of the deciduous dentition.

The pulp canals are wide and tapering and there is no clear demarcation between pulp chamber and root canal. The canals may terminate in an apical delta. Occasionally the canals of lower incisors may be divided into two branches by a mesiodistal wall of dentine.

43

According to G. V. Black (1908), upper deciduous incisors are, on average, 16 mm long, whilst the laterals are slightly shorter. Lower central incisors are, at 14 mm, shorter by a millimetre than the lateral incisors. The canines are the longest deciduous teeth, the uppers being 19 mm and the lowers about 17 mm.

### *The Deciduous Molars* (*Fig.* 30)

As in the permanent dentition the upper molars are three rooted whilst the lower molars have two roots.

The pulp chambers are large in relation to tooth size, and the pulp horns are well developed, particularly in the second molars. From a restorative point of view it is as well to remember that the tip of the pulp horns may be as close as 2 mm from the enamel surface, and thus great care must be taken in the preparation of these teeth if an exposure is to be avoided. Because of the relatively large size of the pulp chamber there is relatively less tooth substance protecting the pulp.

The furcation of the roots is also very much closer to the cervical area of the crown and thus excessive instrumentation of the floor of the pulp chamber may lead to a perforation.

The root canal system is more complicated than in the permanent dentition and roots with two canals often show relatively large interconnecting branches.

Lower molars normally have two root canals in each of the roots, and the mesiobuccal root canal of the upper molars sometimes divides into two. Thus both upper and lower primary molars frequently have four canals.

## ROOT APEX CALCIFICATION

Whilst calcification and cement deposition at the apex of a root continues throughout the life apices can be said to be fully formed at the following ages:

| | |
|---|---|
| Deciduous central and lateral incisors | 2 years |
| Deciduous cuspids and molars | 3 years |
| Permanent first molar | 9 years |
| Permanent central incisors | 10 years |
| Permanent lateral incisor | 11 years |
| Permanent bicuspids | 15 years |
| Permanent second molar | 16–17 years |
| Permanent third molar | 21 years |

REFERENCES

Chapman C. E. (1969) A microscopic study of the apical region of human anterior teeth. *J. Br. Endodont. Soc.* **3**, 52.

Harty F. J., Parkins B. J. and Wengraf A. M. (1970) The success rate of apicectomy. A retrospective study of 1016 cases. *Br. Dent. J.* **129**, 407.

Hess W. and Zurcher F. (1925) *The Anatomy of the Root Canals of the Teeth of the Permanent Dentition and the Anatomy of the Root Canals of the Teeth of the Deciduous Dentition and the First Permanent Molars.* London, Bale, Sons & Danielsson.

Kramer I. R. H. (1960) The vascular architecture of the human dental pulp. *Arch. Oral. Biol.* **2**, 177.

Kuttler Y. (1955) Microscopic investigation of root apexes. *J. Am. Dent. Assoc.* **50**, 544.

Lowman J. V., Burke, R. S. and Pelleu G. B. (1973) Patent accessory canals: Incidence in molar furcation region. *Oral Surg.* **36**, 580.

Meyer W. (1957) Dental anatomy, histology and physiology. *Int. Dent. J.* **7**, 260.


BIBLIOGRAPHY

Davies G. N. and King R. M. (1961) *Dentistry for the Pre-School Child.* Edinburgh, Livingstone.

Ingle J. I. (1965) *Endodontics.* London, Kimpton.

Wheeler R. S. (1974) *Dental Anatomy, Physiology and Occlusion,* 5th ed. Philadelphia, Saunders.

CHAPTER 4

# CAUSES OF PULPAL INJURY
# AND ITS PREVENTION

DURING the past few years the conservation of teeth by endodontic procedures has again become commonplace. However, most dentists realize that these procedures are not always successful and that the healthy living pulp is still the most satisfactory root filling. Thus the conscientious practitioner should take precautions to prevent any form of pulpal injury.

This is not always easy because most operative procedures involve the destruction of tooth substance and the use of restorative materials which may be harmful to the pulp. What saves the patient and the dentist from endless trouble is the excellent recuperative powers of the dental pulp, which, for its size, is probably one of the least delicate organs in the body.

Unfortunately, there is no accurate way of assessing the histopathological state of the pulp by clinical signs and symptoms alone and often a tooth may become non-vital without causing pain. Sometimes a very minor operative procedure may cause a violent reaction, and in these cases one can only assume that pulpal injury is cumulative and that the pulp had already been damaged, by caries or by some other injury, and had reached a stage where it was unable to withstand further stimulation without producing symptoms. Since it is not feasible to know the degree of pulp injury, the only course open to the conscientious practitioner is to heed the work of histopathologists and to keep pulpal stimuli to the absolute minimum compatible with sound operative technique (Morrant, 1974). Thus a review of the causes of pulp damage and the methods used to reduce or prevent these injuries can be considered as the most basic form of endodontic therapy.

The three main causes of pulpal injury are: (1) Dental caries, (2) Injury during operative procedures, (3) Trauma not associated with operative procedures.

## I. DENTAL CARIES

This is still the chief cause of pulpal injury and the response to the advancing carious lesion has been investigated extensively. Whilst there is no universal agreement on the histopathological picture of the pulp under carious attack the following points are generally accepted.

46

As the carious attack is generally a slow process the pulp defends itself efficiently with the formation of a relatively impermeable sclerotic or translucent zone which may be followed by the formation of a dead tract. Secondary dentine may be deposited on the pulp side of the dentinal tubules. These defensive reactions prevent the passage of toxic substances from the carious lesion to the pulp.

*In initial and moderately deep carious lesions* the pulp remains free from bacterial invasion but may show some early inflammatory changes (Brännström and Lind, 1965; Langeland and Langeland, 1968). These changes are easily reversed once the pulp irritant has been removed and the pulp protected with a sedative dressing that seals the dentinal tubules from the oral environment.

In the deep carious lesion the picture begins to change, but even here the pulp remains remarkably healthy even when the thickness of dentine between the pulp and the floor of the carious cavity is very small (Shovelton, 1972). In this study it was shown that where the thickness of dentine between the pulp and the floor of the carious cavity was over 0·8 mm no signs of pulpal inflammation were seen. Considerable pulp inflammation became apparent only when the thickness of remaining dentine was less than 0·3 mm. Bacteria were not found in the pulp until the cavity floor was 0·2 mm or less from the pulp (Shovelton, 1968). Reeves and Stanley (1966) also studied the problem of bacterial invasion of the pulp and concluded that no pathological changes were seen until the secondary dentine itself was involved.

Since the pulp is not invaded by bacteria until late in the carious process how is it that the pulp becomes inflamed? Massler (1967) has suggested that pulp reactions in deep carious lesions are the result of bacterial toxins, and not a direct result of bacterial invasion. He also points out that an inflamed pulp is not necessarily infected.

The other pertinent question is whether the dentine at the base of the deep carious lesion is infected and if so whether the organisms die after the placement of a satisfactory filling. Several workers (Besic, 1943; MacGregor, 1962); and Fisher, 1966, 1969 have shown that organisms remain viable in the dentine for considerable periods of time, but that these are not active in extending the carious process provided that the amount of caries is small and an adequate dressing or filling is placed in the cavity.

It is now generally agreed that certain lining materials such as calcium hydroxide or zinc oxide and eugenol have, at least, a bacteriostatic action (King et al., 1965; Aponte et al., 1966; Fisher, 1969).

### The Management of the Deep Carious Lesion

The management of the very deep cavity has been the subject of considerable disagreement, and the opposing arguments can be summarized by the views held by Sir John Tomes (1859) and G. V. Black (1908). The former stated that, 'It is better that a layer of discoloured dentine should be allowed to remain for the protection of the pulp rather than run the risk of sacrificing the tooth'. G. V. Black suggested that, 'It is better to expose the pulp of a tooth than leave it covered only with softened dentine'. Current research would seem to favour Sir John Tomes' view. Softened dentine should be removed but hard stained dentine can be safely left and covered with a suitable lining material (*see below*).

The question of whether the remaining carious dentine is infected had been studied by Dorfman et al. (1943) who found that the superficial carious dentine was always heavily contaminated with micro-organisms, the middle layers were sometimes infected and the deep layers were nearly always sterile. This was confirmed by Sarnat and Massler (1965). MacGregor et al. (1956) have also shown that the softening of dentine occurs before the dentinal tubules are contaminated by micro-organisms.

It is as well to remember that the object of indirect pulp capping is to protect the pulp from direct bacterial contamination through an actual exposure. Clinically an exposure is recognized by the resultant haemorrhage. However, an exposure may not always be visible because the small blood vessels, the metarterioles and the precapillaries immediately below the odontoblastic layer, may have diameters as small as 8 microns. If these minute blood vessels are severed haemorrhage may not occur and even if it does it will probably be invisible to the naked eye. This type of exposure is often referred to as a *micro-exposure*. Thus, the classical bleeding exposure represents a relatively severe pulp wound (Paterson, 1974a and b).

For this reason and also because accidental carious exposure of the deep carious cavity is always possible it may be prudent if deep cavities are investigated under rubber dam so that the possibility of bacterial contamination is minimized.

The importance of bacterial contamination as a factor influencing the response of the exposed pulp has been demonstrated by Kake-hashi et al. (1965, 1969) and Paterson (1972). In these studies germ-free rats were used and it was shown that the pulp wound healed irrespective of the dressing applied to it. Indeed, even large exposures left untreated healed with very little evidence of pulpal inflammation or necrosis. The materials used for capping the exposures also did not affect the outcome. Paterson (1972) investigated calcium hydroxide, a corticosteroid preparation and ortho-ethoxybenzoic acid (EBA) cement and showed that all materials showed a significant reduction in inflammation and necrosis in the pulps of the germ-free group. This was accompanied by significantly better repair, as manifested by the calcific barrier formation.

The interesting point in the experiment is that teeth exposed and left open to the oral environment in the germ-free rats showed the same degree of calcific repair as the pulps that had been capped with the materials mentioned above.

Clinically an *indirect pulp capping* technique should be used in all cases where a micro-exposure is suspected or where it is considered that the removal of the last vestige of caries will lead to an exposure.

Caries is removed from all areas unlikely to be exposed and the tooth isolated, preferably with rubber dam. The area likely to be exposed is instrumented carefully and all softened dentine removed with a large excavator or a very slowly rotating large round bur. Hard, stained carious dentine is not disturbed but covered with a creamy layer of pulp capping material (*see below*). When set this is reinforced with a further layer of quick setting zinc oxide or zinc phosphate cement onto which the permanent filling can be condensed.

### The Management of the Exposed Vital Pulp

It is possible to conserve an exposed vital pulp by a *direct pulp capping* technique but it must be made quite clear that the chances of success are less than in the indirect technique. If success is to be assured certain criteria must be observed. These are:

1. The pulp exposure must be small, i.e. of no more than about 1 mm².
2. Carious exposures are usually not suitable because the exposure site is inevitably heavily infected and the pulp already invaded by bacteria and probably chronically inflamed.
3. The cavity must be kept free from salivary contamination in order to prevent pulp infection which will lessen the chance of pulp healing.
4. Age plays an important part in the success of the operation. Direct pulp capping is most successful in permanent teeth of young patients probably due to the pulp's rich blood supply and the favourable repair possibilities. However, pulp capping of deciduous teeth is less successful than in young adult's teeth possibly due to rapid and near total involvement of the deciduous pulp in the face of an advancing carious lesion. Massler (1967) states that pulp healing is demonstrably slower in primary than in permanent teeth. He suggests that the open apical foramina of deciduous teeth prevent the rapid calcific response and 'calcific scarring' seen in young permanent teeth in spite of a blood supply that is considerably less than in the deciduous dentition.

49

5. The direct capping of a symptomless tooth has a better chance of success than a tooth that has had specific symptoms. A tooth that has been spontaneously painful without an exciting cause, such as heat, cold or pressure on the pulp due to food packing into the carious cavity, is unlikely to be saved by direct pulp capping alone. Nyborg (1955, 1958) reported a clinical success rate of 86 per cent in teeth with no previous symptoms but this dropped to 46 per cent in teeth with a history of previous pain.

The technique of direct pulp capping differs from the indirect technique because the exposure is usually accompanied by haemorrhage. This is arrested by careful swabbing with the blunt ends of sterile paper points or with cottonwool. The cavity is then irrigated with sterile water or more conveniently with local analgesic solution. Irrigation is necessary to remove traces of blood from the cavity and this prevents tooth staining and also obtains a clean dentine surface onto which the pulp capping material will flow easily and adhere mechanically. The cavity is gently dried with sterile cottonwool rather than a blast of air which might traumatize the exposed pulp and initiate further bleeding. The pulp capping material is flowed onto the exposure and allowed to set before it is protected with a secondary lining of quick setting zinc oxide.

Metal or plastic pulp caps are sometimes advocated for the protection of the pulp from pressure. These were useful when the only available pulp capping materials did not harden quickly or remained soft indefinitely (e.g. calcium hydroxide powder and water). The newer two paste pulp capping materials, e.g. Hydrex* or Dycal†, set very quickly and have a sufficiently high compressive strength to allow the insertion of an even harder lining over them without the risk of forcing the capping material into the pulp.

### Materials used in Pulp Capping

Many different materials have been advocated for both indirect and direct pulp capping but few have stood the test of time.

Ideally the material should have the following properties:
1. Sedative, non-irritating and antiseptic.
2. A good thermal insulator.
3. Able to be applied to the exposed pulp with little or no pressure.
4. Harden rapidly without shrinkage or expansion.

---

*Kerr Manufacturing Co., Romulus, Michigan 48174, U.S.A.
†The L.D. Caulk Co., Milford, Delaware 19963, U.S.A.

5. The physiological response of the pulp should be such that a calcific barrier forms between the material and the vital pulp.

The following materials are in common use:
1. Calcium hydroxide.
2. Corticosteroid-antibiotic compounds.
3. Zinc oxide preparations.
4. Cyanoacrylates.

### 1. Calcium Hydroxide

This material is almost universally used for both direct and indirect pulp capping. It has been extensively investigated and is usually the control for other materials under review.

Nevertheless, its exact mode of action is not understood. Shovelton (1968) suggests that the alkaline properties of the material neutralize the acidity of the softened dentine and may recalcify and harden it. On the other hand, Sciaky and Pisanti (1960) have shown that the calcium ions in the applied calcium hydroxide are not incorporated in the dentine bridge formed beneath the pulp cap.

Evidence seems to favour the view that the softened dentine remaining in indirect pulp capping is remineralized and hardened when this material is used. Mjör et al. (1960) showed this by a radiographic technique and Solomons and Neuman (1960), Sobel (1961) and Eidelman et al. (1965) support this view.

Many studies have been undertaken to compare the efficacy of various materials and in the majority calcium hydroxide has proved superior to other materials. Nyborg (1955, 1958) studied calcium hydroxide and an inert material and found significantly better results with the calcium hydroxide. Shovelton et al. (1971) compared calcium hydroxide, two anti-inflammatory antibiotic materials and zinc oxide with eugenol. Of these the most successful materials in teeth without a history of pain were calcium hydroxide and Ledermix (see below) and when pain had been present the most successful result appeared to be that obtained after using Ledermix paste for 3 days followed by permanent capping with calcium hydroxide. Ledermix paste followed by Ledermix cement gave less successful results.

### 2. Corticosteroid–Antibiotic Preparations

The use of medicaments to eliminate dental pain is not a new concept and oil of cloves alone or in combination with other essential oils has been used for centuries. In 1965 Schroeder suggested the use of a material containing a corticosteroid and a broad spectrum antibiotic as a pulp cap and also as a method of eliminating dental pain.

A typical commercial preparation is 'Ledermix'* which is available in paste and cement form and whose formula consists of the following:

*Paste*
 Triamcinolone acetonide 1 per cent
 Demethylchlortetracycline HCl 3 per cent
  in a water-soluble cream containing triethanolamine, calcium chloride, zinc oxide, sodium sulphate and polyethylene glycol 4000.

*Cement*
 Powder:  Triamcinolone acetonide 0·67 per cent
     Demethylchlortetracycline in a base containing 2 per cent Canada balsam rosin
     Calcium hydroxide
 Liquid 'F'  Eugenol in rectified turpentine oil
 Liquid 'S'  Eugenol.
     Polyethylene glycol in rectified turpentine oil.

The rationale in the use of this medicament is that the steroid will suppress the inflammatory response whilst the antibiotic will inhibit micro-organisms. Presumably the calcium hydroxide is added to promote a dentine bridge across the exposure.

Several clinical trials have been carried out and all agree that the preparation affords relief of symptoms when applied to the exposed pulp of a painful tooth (Ehrmann, 1965; Schroeder, 1965; Allwright and Wong, 1966; Cowan, 1966; Olsen, 1966).

However, controversy exists concerning the action of the material and the resultant histopathological picture, but the most important consideration is the use of the material as a pulp cap and whether a dentine bridge forms at the site of exposure. Studies by Cowan (1966), Olsen (1966), Mjör and Östby (1966), Rowe (1967), Clarke (1968) and Barker and Ehrmann (1969) suggest that a dentine bridge does not form under the material in human teeth, but Schroeder (1965) reported 3 cases where the exposure was bridged by dentine.

Paterson (1974a), in a classic series of experiments, showed that a dentine bridge occurred in the exposed molars of germ-free rats after capping the exposures with various materials including Ledermix. However, the bridge did not form in the control group of normal animals and one must assume that the bridge occurred because of the germ-free conditions rather than because of the materials used. As mentioned before, his experiments reinforce the fact that pulp capping, irrespective of the material used, should be carried out under aseptic conditions to ensure long term success.

It would appear, therefore, that clinically the material is useful for relieving acute pulp pain but evidence has not been presented of its use as a long-term pulp cap.

---

*'Ledermix': Lederle Laboratories–Cyanamid of G.B. Ltd., Bush House, London WC2.

### 3. *Zinc Oxide*

Controversy exists concerning the use of zinc oxide/eugenol as a pulp capping material. Several studies have shown that it is less satisfactory than calcium hydroxide (Glass and Zander, 1949; Weiss and Bjorvatn, 1970; Shovelton et al., 1971; Shovelton, 1972; Nixon and Hannah, 1972).

Massler (1972) has suggested that the failure of zinc oxide as a pulp cap may be due to the significant amount of lead present in commercial or even U.S.P. grades. He suggests that the lead contaminant may injure the pulp, and thus prevent bridge formation.

### 4. *Cyanoacrylates*

The use of isobutyl cyanoacrylate (commercially available as 'Cyanodont'*) as a pulp capping agent has been suggested by Bhaskar et al. (1969) who found the material easy to apply and possessing some haemostatic properties. Both Bhaskar and his colleagues and Berkman et al. (1971) considered the material as effective as calcium hydroxide.

Nixon and Hannah (1972) studied *n*-butyl cyanoacrylate and found that it failed to produce satisfactory dentine barriers and that there was an unsatisfactory pulpal reaction, possibly related to the low pH of the material immediately before polymerization.

It must be emphasized that these investigations are animal studies and the assessment of the material in human teeth has not yet been reported. Its clinical use must therefore be considered experimental.

## II. INJURY DURING OPERATIVE PROCEDURES

Pulp injury can be caused by one or a combination of the following: (1) Injury during tooth preparation; (2) Injury during the débridement; (3) Injury during and after the placement of the restoration.

### 1. *Injury during Tooth Preparation*

During cavity preparation the pulp may be injured by the physical cutting of dentine and by the heat generated by the cutting instrument.

Fish (1932) showed that the cutting of dentinal tubules caused a degeneration of the odontoblastic layer on the pulp surface below the cut area. If the injury was severe then spontaneous haemorrhaging occurred in the body of the pulp. Provided the injury was not severe, secondary dentine formed below the dentinal tubules.

---

*Cyanodont: Specialités Septodont, 29 Rue des Petites Écuries, Paris (10ᵉ).

He also suggested that unless the cut dentinal tubules were sealed from the oral environment and from irritating materials the pulp injury became irreversible.

Whether the pulp recovers from the trauma of dentine cutting depends on the severity of the injury which is, in turn, related to one or more of the following physical factors.

### a. Speed of the Cutting Instrument

From a pulp injury viewpoint 'speed' begins at about 300 r.p.m. At this speed Langeland (1961) found that odontoblastic reaction was minimal. Marsland and Shovelton (1957) reported similar results at speeds of 500 r.p.m.

The greatest amount of odontoblastic damage occurs at speeds up to 50 000 r.p.m. with both belt and turbine driven instruments and the least amount of damage occurs at speeds of 150 000–250 000 r.p.m., provided that a coolant is used (Seltzer and Bender, 1965). The same authors suggest that without water coolant there is no safe speed. However, with sharp burs at 3000 r.p.m. and no coolant there is less damage than there is at ultra-high speed without coolant.

### b. Heat and Pressure

These are considered together because they generally affect the pulp simultaneously. During tooth preparation the cutting instrument generates frictional heat proportional to the pressure with which the instrument is held against the tooth.

Peyton (1955a and b) studied the relationship between rotary speeds, coolants, pressure and temperature rise in teeth *in vitro*. He found that when using a carbide bur without coolant and at a pressure of half a pound, the temperature rise, measured by thermocouples placed in the tooth, was 120° F (49° C). When the pressure was increased to one pound the temperature rose to 175° F (80° C). He also showed that whilst water spray cooling was more effective than air cooling, neither prevented some increase in temperature within the pulp.

Similar results were obtained by Schuchard and Watkins (1960) and Zach and Cohen (1962) who repeated the experiments in *in vivo* conditions. Brännström (1962) considered that increased pressure may result in the displacement of the odontoblastic nuclei.

Cooling during cutting is of paramount importance irrespective of the speed of the cutting instrument. The feeling put forward by some clinicians that it is unnecessary is not substantiated by numerous research studies (Bodecker, 1939; Stanley and Swerdlow, 1960; Morrant, 1969).

Further the quality of the cooling device must be such that the dentine being cut is constantly bathed by the water or water-spray. This is not always possible because most handpieces have a fixed water spray directed at a particular point and the cutting instruments may differ in shape, length and diameter. Thus it is possible for the fixed water spray to be deflected by the instrument or be directed at a point well away from the area being cut. Thus an adjustable spray as fitted to some handpieces is desirable.

### c. Area of Preparation

The area of cut dentine has a bearing on the problem and the more extensive the preparation the more likely it is that the pulp will be injured. One square millimetre of dentine may have 40 000–70 000 dentinal tubules. Zach and Cohen (1958) showed that the pulp damage was roughly proportional to the amount of tooth removed. The volume of cut dentine is also important and preparations with feather margins are less harmful to the pulp than shoulder preparations because the latter have to be cut deep into dentine and are thus closer to the pulp.

In the author's opinion, the current vogue for bonded porcelain restorations has considerably increased the incidence of pulp necrosis. This may be due to the removal of considerable labial or buccal tooth surface in order to accommodate an adequate thickness of porcelain as well as the gold base.

Pinledge preparations are useful in lessening the amount of dentine destruction. However, the preparation of the pinhole with high speed instrumentation should be avoided because the coolant cannot reach the depth of the preparation.

However, a measure of the pulp's resilience may be gauged by the lack of symptoms following the preparation of a tooth for a porcelain jacket crown, where a tooth is denuded of all enamel and a large number of tubules cut in one visit. Patients seldom complain of after pain and the pulp normally recovers from this severe operation. This may be because the temporary crown is usually cemented in place with zinc oxide/eugenol temporary cement which effectively seals the tubules and thus protects the pulp.

### d. The Type and Efficiency of the Cutting Instrument

The efficiency of an instrument depends on its design and on its sharpness. An instrument of large diameter has a higher peripheral speed, at a given r.p.m., than an instrument with a smaller diameter. Because of the higher speed more heat is generated and the pulp may be damaged.

A blunt instrument requires greater pressure and more time to cut a given surface area and both these factors may contribute to further pulp damage.

Peyton (1958) showed that a steel bur produced more heat than carbide or diamond burs irrespective of the method of cooling. Provided the carbide or diamond bur is cooled efficiently the pulp damage is minimal and easily reversible.

### e. Dentine Thickness

Clearly the thinner the dentine layer between the pulp and the floor and walls of the cavity the greater is the likelihood of severe pulp damage, due to pressure, heat and the subsequent effects of drugs and dental materials.

Superficial preparation just into dentine produces only mild pulp irritation which acts as a stimulus resulting in the formation of secondary dentine.

## 2. Injury during Débridement

A pulp may also be damaged whilst the cavity is made ready for the insertion of the permanent restoration.

Formerly it was taught that 'cavity toilet' was an important step in the long term success of the restoration. This consisted of drying the cavity thoroughly with a hot air blast, sterilizing the dentine chemically and then redrying the 'sterile' dentine.

Brännström (1960) has shown that excess dehydration with an air blast causes odontoblastic nucleus displacement. It has also been shown that this dehydration makes the dentine more permeable to any sterilizing agent or filling material placed upon it.

The use of potent sterilizing agents such as phenol, alcohol, thymol, iodine and silver nitrate have been shown to be not only unnecessary for the pulp but harmful. None of these materials are effective in the complete elimination of bacteria from the dentinal tubules. In any event it is now thought that the complete sterilization of dentine is not necessary for any organisms left behind will either die or become ineffective because of the abscence of nutrients within the sealed cavity.

Clinically cavities must be dried before the final insertion of the filling and it is considered that gentle swabbing with cottonwool or a cellulose tissue followed by the light application of warm air is sufficient to produce an acceptable superficial dryness of the dentine (Morrant, 1974).

## 3. Injury during and after the Placement of the Restoration

The pulp may be injured by the toxicity of the restorative material, by the temperature changes during the setting of some materials, by extremes of heat or cold transmitted to the pulp through an inadequately lined filling and also during polishing. Even when the material is fully set the pulp can be affected by microleakage through imperfect margins.

The toxicity of silicate cement is well known and is due to the pH when set and to the presence of minute quantities of arsenic. In spite of certain manufacturers' recommendations composite fillings also require a protective lining in the same way as silicates and conventional or 'filled' methyl methacrylate fillings. The latter may be harmful due to temperature increases during the polymerization reaction.

The pulp must also be protected from thermal changes during eating and thus it is necessary to place an insulating lining between the pulp and the filling, particularly if it is metallic. Of recent years film liners consisting of two separate pastes have become popular because of their ease of application and also because it was realized that liners of relatively small compressive strengths were sufficiently strong for amalgam condensation. However, these materials do not have sufficient bulk to protect the pulp from thermal shock and thus in deep cavities they must be reinforced with an over-lining able to give adequate thermal insulation.

The polishing of amalgam may also cause problems due to temperature rise and should be carried out slowly and, if possible, under water spray.

*Microleakage* is also said to be a factor in pulp injury both under amalgam and under tooth coloured filling materials. Phillips (1965) demonstrated the marginal leakage around newly placed amalgams by radio-isotope studies. He suggested that the routine use of copal ether varnish over the dentine and enamel walls would prevent this microleakage. The problem is probably academic with regard to amalgam, for as Pickard and Gayford (1965) pointed out amalgam fillings corrode after a few weeks and provide an efficient marginal seal.

Microleakage is more relevant in autopolymerizing restorations where the high coefficient of thermal expansion results in a distinct space between the filling and the cavity walls. To a lesser degree the problem is similar with the composite resins. To date no solution is available in these instances but it is possible that the development of acid-etch technique may overcome the difficulty.

## III. TRAUMA NOT ASSOCIATED WITH OPERATIVE PROCEDURES

The pulp may be damaged in various ways not associated with caries or with operative procedures.

In a book of this size it is not possible to deal, at length, with these topics nor discuss the underlying histopathology. Nevertheless, the management of such traumatic lesions is important and will be discussed briefly.

Trauma may be accidental, physiological, iatrogenic or caused by the patient.

### 1. *Accidental Trauma*

If the trauma is severe enough the apical blood vessels are severed or crushed and the pulp becomes necrotic. This may occur without any other visible signs of injury and the treatment in such cases is conventional root therapy.

If the injury is less severe the pulp reacts, as in any other connective tissue, by an inflammatory response. After an acute phase the pulp may develop a chronic inflammation and a certain amount of fibrous repair occurs. The tooth becomes symptomless but the pulp is unable to withstand further injury as well as previously and a subsequent relatively minor stimulus may result in a flare up which may lead to pulp death.

Alternatively the odontoblasts in the inflamed pulp may react by elaborating large quantities of dentine and the root canal becomes calcified. This filling in of the pulp chamber begins in the coronal area and proceeds apically, and for this reason traumatized teeth must be checked radiographically frequently and root filled conventionally lest part of the canal is obliterated. In fact the entire canal is seldom calcified and the apical third may remain patent although the pulp in this area may have degenerated. This portion may become infected but, because the coronal and cervical two-thirds are blocked, conventional root therapy becomes difficult, if not impossible, and root therapy by surgical means is the only way of saving the tooth.

The above instances can occur either with or without crown or root fracture. The management of root fracture is discussed in Chapter 11.

The management of crown fractures will depend on the site of the fracture and the age of the patient.

*Fractures of the enamel* alone generally require no treatment except for the smoothing of any sharp edges to prevent irritation of the soft tissues. In young patients the pulp may have to be protected from thermal stimuli. A temporary cellophane crown is filled with a quick setting zinc oxide and placed on the tooth for some two to three weeks.

The use of an acid-etch/composite technique may provide a more satisfactory and aesthetically pleasing solution to this problem (*see next page*).

*In the coronal fracture with dentine involvement* the pulp must be protected because the dentinal tubules in freshly exposed dentine are patent and the pulp's defence mechanism has not had time to come into effect as it does under the much slower carious attack. The exposed dentine may be protected by a quick setting zinc oxide/eugenol cement held in position with a celluloid or metal crown form. It is also possible to provide a more permanent and aesthetically pleasing protective covering by an acid-etch/composite technique. As soon as possible after the fracture the exposed dentine is dried with cottonwool and a thin layer of calcium hydroxide flowed onto the exposed dentine and allowed to harden.

The enamel surrounding the fracture is etched and the missing portion of tooth restored with a composite fashioned in a cellophane form. This technique holds the calcium hydroxide lining in place, seals the exposed tubules from oral fluid contamination, looks better than the zinc oxide/eugenol crown form restoration and lasts considerably longer.

*In coronal fractures with pulp involvement* three possible courses of treatment may be given, viz. pulp capping, pulpotomy or conventional root therapy.

*Pulp capping* is seldom successful unless the exposure is very small for the reasons given on p. 49.

*Pulpotomy* is more successful than pulp capping and is particularly useful in teeth with incompletely developed apices. This has been described on p. 182.

*Pulp extirpation* is indicated in teeth where the exposure is more than 1 mm², where there has been a history of pain (as opposed to sensitivity to temperature changes) or where the exposure occurred more than 24 hours previously.

As stated before a visible exposure is a relatively severe pulp wound and this, coupled with the trauma sustained by the tooth, usually results in irreversible pulp damage necessitating pulp extirpation.

*Fractured cusps* in posterior teeth are not always easy to discover and sometimes give rise to indefinite clinical symptoms. The patient usually complains of an infrequent pain whilst chewing, which is particularly noticeable as the teeth are brought out of occlusion. A useful diagnostic aid consists of placing a section of rubber (cut from an analgesic cartridge plunger) between opposing teeth and asking the patient to close. The fractured tooth will often give a painful reaction as the teeth are brought out of occlusion. Confirmation of the fracture may be obtained by isolating the tooth with a rubber dam, and drying and painting it with a dye such as methylene blue. After a few minutes the dye is washed off with water and the tooth redried. The dye usually penetrates the fracture line and makes it visible. Treatment will depend on the extent of the injury.

## 2. *Physiological Trauma*

The pulp is affected by attrition which can be defined as the slow, physiological wearing away of the enamel, and ultimately of the dentine, during mastication. Attrition is common in individuals whose diet contains coarse foods, e.g. Australian aborigines. In Western society the most common cause of attrition is, probably, bruxism which takes place during sleep or unconsciously during the day.

The process is slow and the pulp protects itself by the formation of secondary dentine which is deposited in greater amounts on the roof and the floor of the pulp chamber. Thus the pulp chamber 'shrinks' more in the longitudinal axis of the tooth than in the mesio-distal or buccolingual planes. The pulp horns in molars do not recede as quickly as the main body of the pulp and their exposure during cavity preparation must be avoided.

The same anatomical changes occur as an individual ages. The pulp itself becomes less vascular and thus less able to overcome relatively minor traumata and necrosis may occur. As has been mentioned in Chapter 3, access to such constricted canals may be difficult and the access cavity has to be designed with greater care so as not to destroy enamel and dentine unnecessarily.

*Pulp stones or denticles* may occur in pulps that have been mildly irritated over a long period of time. These deposits of amorphous calcific material occur around the pulpal vessels in an otherwise normal tooth. If root therapy should become necessary in such a tooth the access cavity must be large enough to allow the removal of the stone *in toto* prior to the débridement of the remainder of the canal.

*Malocclusion* and the traumatic occlusion of individual teeth have sometimes been blamed for the necrosis of a pulp. In fact there are no conclusive studies that show a relationship between traumatic occlusion and histopathological changes in the pulp.

Rocking and jiggling a tooth over long periods leads to a thickening of the periodontal ligament rather than pulp changes and the pulp may then become involved because of the periodontal problems that arise (Ramfjord and Ash, 1966).

The reason why pulp involvement is uncommon is that the dentition's defence mechanism is good and the patient will either train himself not to chew on the affected tooth or the tooth will move relatively rapidly out of occlusion. A third possibility is that the involved cusp will fracture.

Very minor and longstanding occlusal trauma, however, may lead to calcification of a large part of the pulp and very rarely to pulp necrosis.

## 3. Iatrogenic Trauma

Iatrogenic trauma may be caused by operative procedures (see p. 53), by orthodontic or periodontic treatment and by pulp injury during surgery. Radiation therapy for carcinoma of the oral cavity or the neck may also affect the pulps of teeth.

### Orthodontic Treatment

Mild forces applied to teeth cause a pulp hyperaemia which is reversible once the force is removed (Anstendig and Kronman, 1972). It has also been noted that the teeth of patients undergoing orthodontic treatment are more sensitive to thermal changes.

Severe force to obtain a rapid tooth movement, particularly in an apical direction, results in partial or total pulp degeneration in the same way as a blow to the tooth.

Orthodontic movement may cause apical or root resorption without apparently affecting pulp vitality.

It is as well to remember that pulp injury is a cumulative process and conservative procedures in teeth undergoing orthodontic treatment should be carried out with great care because the pulp may not be able to withstand the extra irritation caused by the conservative treatment. Frequent examination of the dentition of children undergoing orthodontic treatment is imperative so that any carious lesions are detected and treated early in order to keep the preparations as small and as shallow as possible.

### Periodontal Disease

The pulp may be injured during periodontal procedures by the severance of blood vessels entering the pulp through lateral canals. Sometimes these canals carry blood vessels of greater diameter than the vessels entering through the apical foramen (Kramer, 1960) and their severance leads to pulp atrophy and degeneration. The exposure of fresh dentine following periodontal treatment presents problems of management because the tooth may become sensitive to thermal changes which are difficult to control. Such sensitive areas are often treated by desensitizing agents which must be carefully chosen lest they act as pulp irritants. Drugs such as formalin, zinc chloride, silver nitrate, phenol and sodium fluoride should be avoided because they may enter the pulp through lateral canals and cause injury. The repeated use of a silicone varnish such as 'Tresiolan'* affords relief from this condition without apparent pulp damage.

Reports on the effect of ultrasonic scaling on the pulp are conflicting. Hansen and Nielsen (1956) found that some interference occurred with both amelogenesis and dentinogenesis. Seltzer and

Bender (1965) state that, 'Many investigators have reported that the use of ultrasonic instruments on the teeth of dogs, monkeys and humans caused no more damage to the pulp than did rotary instruments.'

The relationship of periodontal disease and endodontics has been considered fully in Chapter 10.

*Surgical procedures* may lead to pulpal injury either adjacent or some distance away from the operating site by interference with the blood supply. Sometimes due to poor surgical access a wrong root may be unintentionally damaged during apicectomy.

### Radiation Therapy

The pulps of patients receiving radiation treatment may be affected if the site of malignancy is in the oral cavity or in the neck. The odontoblasts may become necrotic and the pulp fibrosed. The dentine and enamel becomes extremely brittle and the teeth are caries prone due to a decrease in salivary flow. Because of the risk of bone necrosis non-vital teeth in such patients should be conventionally root filled rather than extracted.

## REFERENCES

Allwright W. C. and Wong A. P. C. (1966) Corticosteroid and antibiotic combination in the treatment of pulpitis: a clinical trial in Hong Kong. *Dent. Pract. Dent. Rec.* **16**, 168.

Anstendig H. S. and Kronman J. H. (1972) A histologic study of pulpal reaction to orthodontic tooth movement in dogs. *Angle Orthod.* **42**, 50.

Aponte A. J., Hartsook J. T. and Crowley M. C. (1966) Indirect pulp capping success verified. *J. Dent. Child.* **33**, 164.

Barker B. C. W. and Ehrmann E. H. (1969) Human pulp reactions to a glutocorticosteroid antibiotic compound. *Aust. Dent. J.* **14**, 104.

Berkman M. D., Cucolo F. A., Levin, M. P. and Brunelle L. J. (1971) Pulpal response to isobutyl cyanoacrylate in human teeth. *J. Am. Dent. Assoc.* **83**, 140.

Besic F. C. (1943) The fate of bacteria sealed in dental cavities. *J. Dent. Res.* **22**, 349.

Bhaskar S. N., Cutnight D. E., Boyers R. C. and Margetis P. M. (1969) Pulp capping with isobutyl cyanoacrylate. *J. Am. Dent. Assoc.* **79**, 640.

Black G. V. (1908). *A Work on Operative Dentistry*, Vol. II. Chicago, Medico-Dental Publishing.

Bodecker C. F. (1939) Demonstration of possible ill effects of heat on the pulp caused by rapid operative technic. *J. Am. Dent. Assoc.* **26**, 527.

Brännström M. (1960) Dentinal and pulpal response. III, Application of an air stream to exposed dentine—Long observation periods. *Acta Odontol. Scand.* **18**, 235.

---

*'Tresiolan' Espe GMBH. Seefeld Oberban, West Germany.

Brännström M. (1962) Dentinal and pulpal response. VI, Some experiments with heat and pressure illustrating the movement of odontoblasts into the dentinal tubules. *Oral Surg.* **15**, 203.

Brännström M. and Lind P. O. (1965) Pulpal response to early dental caries. *J. Dent. Res.* **44**, 1045.

Clarke N. G. (1968) The response of human pulp to corticosteroid tetracycline cement. *Dent. Pract. Dent. Rec.* **18**, 236.

Cowan A. (1966) Treatment of exposed vital pulps with a corticosteroid antibiotic agent. *Br. Dent. J.* **120**, 521.

Dorfman A., Stephan R. M. and Muntz J. A. (1943) In vitro studies on sterilization of carious dentin. II, Extent of infection in carious lesions. *J. Am. Dent. Assoc.* **30**, 1901.

Ehrmann E. H. (1965) The effect of triamcinolone with tetracycline on the dental pulp and apical periodontium. *J. Prosthet. Dent.* **15**, 144.

Eidelman E., Finn S. B. and Koulourides T. (1965), Remineralization of carious dentine treated with calcium hydroxide. *J. Dent. Child.* **32**, 218.

Fish E. W. (1932) *An Experimental Investigation of Enamel, Dentine and the Dental Pulp.* London, John Bale, Sons & Danielsson.

Fisher F. J. (1966) The viability of micro-organisms in carious dentine beneath amalgam restorations. *Br. Dent. J.* **121**, 413.

Fisher F. J. (1969) The effect of a calcium hydroxide/water paste on micro-organisms in carious dentine. *Br. Dent. J.* **133**, 19.

Glass R. L. and Zander H. A. (1949) Pulp healing. *J. Dent. Res.* **28**, 97.

Hansen L. S. and Nielsen A. G. (1956) Comparison of tissue response to rotary and ultrasonic dental cutting procedures. *J. Am. Dent. Assoc.* **52**, 131.

Kakehashi S., Stanley H. R. and Fitzgerald R. J. (1965) The effects of surgical exposures of dental pulps in germ-free and conventional laboratory rats. *Oral Surg.* **20**, 340.

Kakehashi S., Stanley H. R. and Fitzgerald R. (1969) The exposed germ-free pulp: Effects of topical corticosteroid medication and restoration. *Oral Surg.* **27**, 60.

King J. B., Crawford J. J. and Lindahl R. L. (1965) Indirect pulp capping: A bacteriologic study of deep carious dentine in human teeth. *Oral Surg.* **20**, 663.

Kramer I. R. H. (1960) The vascular architecture of the human dental pulp. *Arch. Oral Biol.* **2**, 177.

Langeland K. (1961) Tissue changes incident to cavity preparation: An evaluation of some dental engines. *Acta Odontol. Scand.* **19**, 397.

Langeland K. and Langeland L. K. (1968) Indirect capping and the treatment of deep carious lesions. *Int. Dent. J.* **18**, 326.

MacGregor A. B. (1962) The extent and distribution of acid in carious dentine. *Proc. R. Soc. Med.* **55**, 1063.

MacGregor A. B., Marsland E. A. and Batty I. (1956) Experimental studies of dental caries. I, The relation of bacterial invasion to softening of the dentine. *Br. Dent. J.* **101**, 230.

Marsland E. A. and Shovelton D. S. (1957) The effect of cavity preparation on the human dental pulp. *Br. Dent. J.* **102**, 213.

Massler M. (1967) Preventive endodontics: vital pulp therapy. *Dent. Clin. North Am.* p. 663.

Massler M. (1972) Therapy conducive to healing of the human pulp. *Oral Surg.* **34**, 122.

Mjör I. A. and Östby N. B. (1966) Experimental investigations on the effect of Ledermix on normal pulps. *J. Oral Ther. Pharmac.* **2**, 367.

Mjör I. A., Quigley M. B. and Finn S. B. (1960) Microchanges in sound human dentine. *J. Dent. Res.* **39**, 715.

Morrant G. A. (1969) Reaction of the dental tissues to cavity preparation with ultra-high-speed rotary instruments. M.D.S. Thesis, University of London.

Morrant G. A. (1974) Preservation of the pulp. In: Harty F. J. and Roberts D. H. (ed.), *Restorative Procedures for the Practising Dentist.* Bristol, Wright.

Nixon G. S. and Hannah C. McD. (1972) *N*-Butyl cyanoacrylate as a pulp capping agent. *Br. Dent. J.* **133**, 14.

Nyborg H. (1955) Healing processes in the pulp on capping: A morphological study. *Acta Odontol. Scand.* **13**, Suppl. 16.

Nyborg H. (1958) Capping of the pulp: The processes involved in their outcome. A report of the follow-ups of a clinical series. *Odontol. Tidskr.* **66**, 293.

Olsen P. (1966) Further experience with triamcinolone-demethylchlortetracycline for conservative endodontic treatment. *J. Can. Dent. Assoc.* **32**, 522.

Paterson R. C. (1972) Bacterial contamination and the response of the exposed rat molar pulp. *J. Dent. Res.* **51**, 1235.

Paterson R. C. (1974a) The effect of various materials on the exposed molar pulps of conventional and germ-free rats. Ph.D. Thesis, University of London.

Paterson R. C. (1974b) Management of the deep cavity. *Br. Dent. J.* **137**, 250.

Peyton F. A. (1955a) Evaluation of dental handpieces for high speed operations. *J. Am. Dent. Assoc.* **50**, 383.

Peyton F. A. (1955b) Temperature rise in teeth developed by rotating instruments. *J. Am. Dent. Assoc.* **50**, 629.

Peyton F. A. (1958) Effectiveness of water coolants with rotary cutting instruments. *J. Am. Dent. Assoc.* **56**, 664.

Phillips R. W. (1965) New concepts in materials used for restorative dentistry. *J. Am. Dent. Assoc.* **70**, 652.

Pickard H. M. and Gayford J. J. (1965) Leakage at the margins of amalgam restorations. *Br. Dent. J.* **119**, 69.

Ramfjord S. P. and Ash M. (1966) *Occlusion.* Philadelphia, Saunders, p. 150.

Reeves R. and Stanley H. R. (1966) The relationship of bacterial penetration and pulpal pathosis in carious teeth. *Oral Surg.* **22**, 59.

Rowe A. H. R. (1967) Reaction of the rat molar pulp to various materials. *Br. Dent. J.* **122**, 291.

Sarnat H. and Massler M. (1965) Microstructure of active and arrested dentinal caries. *J. Dent. Res.* **44**, 1389.

Schroeder A. (1965) Konservative Pulpitistherapie und direkte Uber-kuppany. *Zahnaerztl. Prax.* **16**, 73.

Schuchard A. and Watkins C. (1960) Temperature response to increased rotational speeds. *J. Dent. Res.* **39**, 738.

Sciaky I. and Pisanti S. (1960) Localization of calcium placed over amputated pulps in dogs' teeth. *J. Dent. Res.* **39**, 1128.

Seltzer S. and Bender I. B. (1965) *The Dental Pulp: Biologic Considerations in Dental Procedures.* Philadelphia, Lippincott.

Shovelton D. S. (1968) A study of deep carious dentine. *Int. Dent. J.* **18**, 392.

Shovelton D. S. (1972) The maintenance of pulp vitality. *Br. Dent. J.* **133**, 95.

Shovelton D. S., Friend L. A., Kirk E. E. J. and Rowe A. H. R. (1971) The efficacy of pulp capping materials: A comparative trial. *Br. Dent. J.* **130**, 385.

Sobel A. E. (1961) Remineralization of bones and teeth. *Int. Dent. J.* **11**, 363.

Solomons C. C. and Neuman W. F. (1960) On the mechanisms of calcification: The remineralization of dentin. *J. Biol. Chem.* **235**, 2502.

Stanley H. R. and Swerdlow H. (1960) Biological effects of various cutting methods in cavity preparation: The part pressure plays in pulpal response. *J. Am. Dent. Assoc.* **61**, 450.

Tomes Sir John (1859) *A System of Dental Surgery.* London, Churchill.

Weiss M. B. and Bjorvatn K. (1970) Pulp capping in deciduous and newly erupted permanent teeth of monkeys. *Oral Surg.* **29**, 769.

Zach L. and Cohen G. (1958) Biology of high speed rotary operative dental procedures. I, Correlation of tooth volume removal and pulpal pathology *J. Dent. Res.* **37**, 67.

Zach L. and Cohen G. (1962) Thermogenesis of operative techniques. Comparison of four methods. *J. Prosthet. Dent.* **12**, 977.

CHAPTER 5

# BASIC INSTRUMENTATION IN ENDODONTICS

THE first instruments made specifically for use within the root canal were designed to remove pulp tissue and not to shape the canal walls. These were essentially barbed broaches and Fauchard (1746) described such an instrument which he made from a piece of annealed piano wire, tempered, cut into suitable lengths and mounted on a handle. The barbs were cut with a sharp knife and these he described as 'small beards, looking towards the handle of the instrument'.

The realization that the whole of the pulp cavity had to be cleaned and shaped in order to receive a hermetic root filling is a relatively modern concept and it was not until about 1875 that instruments, other than barbed broaches, began to be manufactured commercially.

Nowadays the endodontist has at his disposal a number of different instruments but he may fail to appreciate their limitations and function. Each group of instruments has a specific purpose which normally cannot be carried out by a different instrument. For example, a reamer is designed to bore a circular hole and cannot be used efficiently as a file. A barbed broach is admirable for the gross removal of pulp tissue but useless in smoothing canal walls.

The contention by some that the débridement and preparation of the entire pulp cavity can be done with one type of instrument alone is incorrect and the conscientious endodontist should have at his disposal, and know how to use, every tool available to him.

The following instruments are readily available and commonly used:

1. Broaches, both smooth and barbed.
2. Reamers.
3. Files:
   *a.* 'K' type
   *b.* Hedstroem
   *c.* Rat-tail.
4. Engine operated instruments.
   *a.* Conventional instruments used in a conventional handpiece:
      i. Burs
      ii. Engine reamers
      iii. Root canal spiral or Lentulo fillers.
   *b.* Specially designed instruments used in a reciprocating handpiece.

5. Auxiliary instruments:
  *a.* Safety devices and rubber dam
  *b.* Measuring stops, gauges and stands
  *c.* Instruments for the retrieval of broken instruments
  *d.* Instruments used in filling root canals.
6. Instruments and equipment for storage and sterilization.
7. Standardized instruments.

## I. BROACHES

These are available as either smooth or barbed (*Fig.* 31). *Smooth broaches* are not widely used but are useful as pathfinders in curved fine canals because of their flexibility and fine diameter. They are

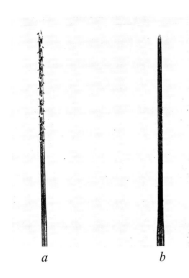

*Fig.* 31. Both barbed and smooth broaches are manufactured from soft steel wire. The barbed broach (*a*) is useful for the gross removal of pulp tissue from the root canal. The smooth broach (*b*) is used mainly to demonstrate pulp exposure and as a pathfinder in curved canals.

*a*    *b*

made from smooth, generally round tapered wire, which neither enlarges nor damages the canal walls. These instruments are also useful in demonstrating pulp exposures and fine root canal openings and are available mounted on handles or as blanks for attachment to a broach holder.

*Barbed broaches* are made from soft steel wire of varying diameters, and the barbs formed by cutting into the metal and forcing the cut portions away from the shaft so that the tip of the barb points towards the handle. The cuts are made eccentrically around the shaft so that it is not weakened excessively at any one point.

Barbed broaches are used mainly for the removal of vital pulp tissue from root canals. They are also useful in the removal of

67

gross debris such as necrotic tissue, cottonwool dressings, paper points and loosely packed gutta percha cones. Occasionally they may prove useful in the removal of a fractured reamer or file.

Provided the instrument is loose within the canal and the barbs used to engage soft tissue only, the risk of fracture or root perforation is minimal. However, as soon as a barbed broach is wedged against the dentine walls the barbs, being of relatively soft metal, flatten against the shaft. When an attempt is made to remove the instrument from the canal the sharp barb tips dig into the canal wall and resist its withdrawal very effectively. Considerable force may be necessary to free the jammed instrument and there is a risk of either fracturing the shaft of the instrument or at least some of the individual delicate barbs. For this reason this instrument should never be used to shape canal walls.

Barbed broaches are used in the 'Giromatic system' and are discussed on p. 76.

## II. REAMERS (*Fig.* 32)

Reamers are made by twisting tapering lengths of wire which have a triangular or square cross section to form an instrument with sharp cutting edges along the spiral. Because of the difficulty of manufacturing fine wire with triangular sections the smaller instruments (sizes 15–50) are usually made from wire of square cross section. The point is sharpened to better penetrate the root canal, and also to lead the instrument into and past any constrictions within the canal. The sharpened point has disadvantages and can lead to ledge formation and to perforations particularly in curved roots (*Fig.* 33). Luks (1959) has described the tip as a 'spear point' and pointed out that few operators realize that it is an extremely active cutting surface.

Ledge formation and root perforation can be prevented by recalling the anatomy of the canal to be instrumented and pre-bending the instrument so that it follows its curvature without impinging on the canal walls. As a further precaution the sharp tip may be blunted with a carborundum disc.

Reamers are used to enlarge and shape an irregularly shaped canal into a cavity of round cross section. They cut primarily at their point and can enlarge the canal only slightly more than their own diameter. The method of use can be likened to the winding of a watch. The instrument is placed in the root canal and wound clockwise through half a turn so that the cutting edges bite into the dentine. The reamer is then unwound by a quarter of a turn and withdrawn. In this way the walls are shaved and dentine cuttings removed from the root canal.

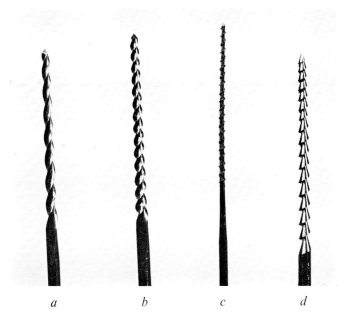

a      b      c      d

*Fig.* 32. Instruments used to cleanse and shape the root canal: *a*, Reamer; *b*, 'K' type file; *c*, Rat-tail file; *d*, Hedstroem file.

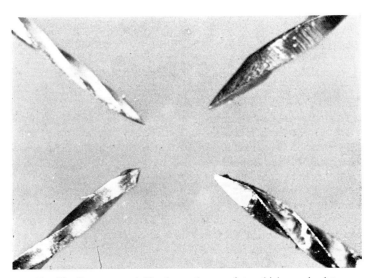

*Fig.* 33. Reamers and files have sharp points which can lead to ledge formation and/or perforation, particularly in curved roots.

In practice reamers are only useful in near round canals. Oval canals have to be filed if the débridement is to be successful. As most root canals are round in their apical 3–4 mm and oval elsewhere it is necessary to ream the apical portion and file the remainder of the canal.

## III. FILES

There are three types of file (or rasp): (1) The 'K' type; (2) The Hedstroem; (3) The rat-tail.

As the name implies these instruments are used with a filing rather than a reaming action and are useful in smoothing and cleaning the walls of an oval or eccentrically shaped root canal. They can enlarge a canal to a size considerably larger than their own diameter.

### 1. The 'K' Type Files (Fig. 32)

These are made in the same way as reamers but have a much tighter spiral thus increasing the number of cutting edges per centimetre. They can be used with a reaming action but because of the increased number of spirals are easily wedged against the dentine walls of the root canal and may fracture if undue force is used.

When manipulated with a filing action they effectively remove dentine and debris from the canal walls. The dentine chips and debris should always be removed from the flutes of the instrument before they are re-inserted in the canals.

Because of the possibility of using these instruments both as a file and as a reamer many practitioners limit their armamentarium to these instruments alone.

### 2. The Hedstroem File (Fig. 32)

These instruments, sometimes called 'root canal rasps', are made by machining steel blanks and so forming tapered instruments composed of a series of cones. The tip is sharpened and may perforate the wall of a curved root. The cone edges are extremely sharp and in a much tighter spiral than the reamer or 'K' type file.

The importance of flexibility in root canal instruments has been stressed by many endodontists and Luks (1959) feels that the flexibility of the shaft is more important than its thickness. Harty and Stock (1974a and b) have found that the Hedstroem file was four times less stiff than either the reamer or the 'K' type file. Thus, because of its flexibility this instrument is admirable for negotiating fine, curved canals.

Because of the method of manufacture the instrument is delicate and easily broken if wedged against the canal walls and then twisted.

70

Therefore, it should be used with a filing or planing action only. As the Hedstroem file has sharp cutting edges it is useful in the retrieving of instruments fractured within the root canal (*see* p. 215).

### 3. *The Rat-tail File (Fig.* 32)

These instruments resemble barbed broaches in that spikes are cut into the shaft and project with their tip towards the handle. These spikes are smaller and more numerous than in a barbed broach. The instrument is normally tapered and only available in the smaller sizes (Nos. 15 to 40). The steel from which rat-tailed files are made is soft, and it can therefore negotiate curved canals easily. The tip of the instrument is rounded and for this reason and also because the metal is relatively soft, root perforation during instrumentation is rare. It is used with a push-pull action and cuts effectively on the pull stroke. Unfortunately the instrument is not available in standardized sizes and by its very action leaves an irregular and rough root canal.

## IV. ENGINE OPERATED INSTRUMENTS AND BURS

These fall into two categories: (1) Conventional instruments and burs used in a conventional handpiece; (2) Specially designed root canal instruments used in a reciprocating handpiece.

### 1. *Conventional Instruments and Burs used in a Conventional Handpiece*

Access into the pulp chamber is obtained with high speed and conventional burs. The importance of access cavity outline has been discussed in Chapter 3. The operation is usually carried out in two stages.

Firstly an access cavity of correct outline should be cut just into dentine. This should be carried out without the use of rubber dam which may obscure anatomical landmarks and hide the true angulation of the tooth and this, in turn, may lead to accidental perforation of the crown or the root.

Next, the rubber dam is placed in position, the field disinfected and the roof of the pulp chamber removed with a slowly rotating round bur. High speed instrumentation and fissure burs should not be used for this stage as the use of the former lessens tactile sense and fissure burs may be advanced too far and damage the normally smooth surface of the floors and walls of the pulp chamber. Visibility, particularly in posterior teeth, may be limited and this can be improved by using long shank burs or conventional burs in a miniature head handpiece (*Fig.* 34).

71

*b. Engine Reamers*

The use of engine operated reamers or other cutting instruments within the root canal is a very dangerous operation because tactile sense is lost and it is very easy to deviate from the canal pathway and perforate the root. There are, however, specially designed reamers which, *on rare occasions*, may be useful in root canal instrumentation. Such an occasion may occur when a portion of an instrument is fractured deep within the root canal and a channel has to be formed so that the broken instrument may be retrieved.

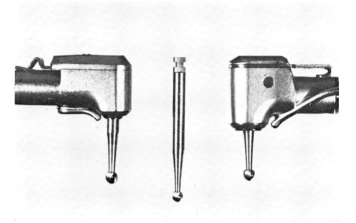

*Fig.* 34. The use of long shank burs or of normal sized burs in a miniature head handpiece improves visibility. The longer bur is also useful in removing the roof of a pulp chamber that has receded away from the occlusal or incisal surface.

Two such special reamers are the *Gates* and the *Peeso* types (*Fig.* 35). The former has a bud-shaped cutting point mounted on a rigid fine shaft which is attached to a latch-type bur shank. The advantage of the Gates reamer lies in its blunt but fine tip which acts as a pathfinder within the root canal without damaging the walls or creating false pathways.

The instrument should be used in a slowly rotating handpiece and removed frequently from the canal, which should be irrigated to wash out dentine chips and also to cool the root surface.

The Peeso-type engine operated reamer is less useful and more dangerous in use than the Gates drill because it resembles a twist drill with a sharpened point and this can only lead to a root perforation. The instrument is really only useful in enlarging a reasonably wide canal in order to prepare the root for a cast metal post-retained restoration.

Conventional round, bud, flame and blunt tipped tapered fissure burs are sometimes advocated for use within the pulp cavity and these should be confined to gaining access to the pulp chamber. Sometimes a flame bur is useful in enlarging the orifice of a very fine root canal in order to make it easier to identify and instrument.

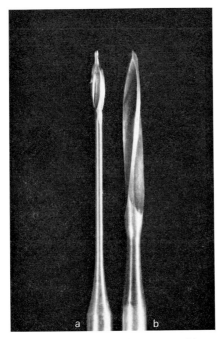

*Fig.* 35. The use of engine operated reamers and burs within the root canal is fraught with danger because of the loss of tactile sense and the risk of root perforation. If a canal has to be reamed in this manner the Gates reamer (*a*) is preferred because the fine but blunt tip acts as a pathfinder without the risk of perforation. The Peeso reamer (*b*) is sometimes useful in removing gutta-percha root fillings in post-retained restorations.

*c. Root Canal, Spiral or Lentulo Fillers (Fig. 36)*

These instruments are normally made from fine wire which is twisted to form a tapered spiral and attached to a bur shank. As the name implies they are used to fill a root canal with paste medicament or with root canal sealer and this they do very efficiently. However, when engine operated they are dangerous because they are liable to become wedged against the canal walls and fracture.

An alternative, and much safer, method of transferring pastes and sealers into the root canal is by means of a reamer two sizes smaller than that used to finally prepare the canal. The shaft of the reamer is marked with the length to which the root canal has been prepared. Paste or sealer is picked up on the reamer and introduced into the canal to the correct level. The paste is then deposited on the canal walls by turning the reamer in an *anti-clockwise* direction. In this way a controlled amount of sealer is deposited within the root canal with no danger of instrument fracture, or of forcing sealer through the apical foramen.

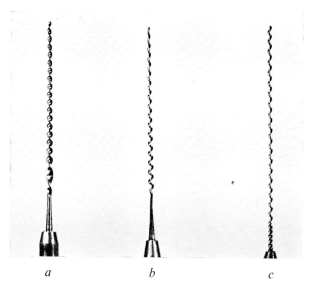

*a*                    *b*                    *c*

*Fig.* 36. Spiral root fillers: (*a*) The Hawes-Neos type is preferred because it is manufactured from a rectangular blade of metal and is therefore stronger than the conventional round wire filler (*b*) or the 'Micro-Mega' filler (*c*).

As well as being delicate, and thus prone to fracture, engine operated spiral fillers may carry too much material into the root canal which may be forced into the periapical tissues by the forward pressure created by the rotary action of the filler (*Fig.* 37).

If spiral fillers are to be used at all they should be selected carefully and used with caution. Some root fillers are safer in use than others. Two such instruments are the 'Hawes-Neos' type* and the 'Micro-Mega'†. The former is manufactured from a rectangular blade of metal and is less likely to fracture because it has a greater cross-section and is therefore stronger than fine wire (Tidmarsh, 1975).

---

*'Hawes-Neos New Type' root filler: 6925 Gentillino, Lugano 3, Switzerland.

†'Micro-Mega' Spiral fillers: Micro-Mega S.A., 5–12 Rue du Tunnel, Besançon 25006, France.

The Micro-Mega filler has a safety mechanism consisting of a tight spiral at the point where the wire shaft joins the bur shank. In this way if the working spiral should jam within the root canal it will fracture, not within the root canal, but at the safety point which normally lies well outside the canal. If the instrument is not jammed tightly within the canal it may be possible to grasp the fractured end with artery forceps and either unwind the spiral from the canal or remove it by pulling in an incisal or occlusal direction.

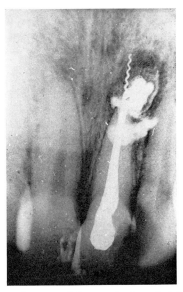

*Fig.* 37. Over-zealous use of the round wire spiral filler has forced sealer and the instrument itself through the apical foramen where it has fractured.

Irrespective of the type of filler used it should never be inserted into the canal whilst rotating. It is safer to mark the shaft of the filler at the calculated root canal length, load the filler with paste or sealer and insert it into the root canal, to the correct level, *with the engine stationary*. The engine is started and at the same time the filler is gently withdrawn. In this way it is unlikely that the filler will jam and fracture.

Generally spiral fillers carry too much sealer into the canal and, indeed, tend to concentrate the material in the apical region of the canal. This excess material must be removed because, on insertion of the obturating gutta percha or silver point, it is possible to force the excess material through the apical foramen. Removal of the excess sealer from the root canal is carried out by re-inserting a dry filler to the correct level, again with the engine stationary. The engine is activated to rotate in an *anti-clockwise* direction and, at the same time, the filler is slowly withdrawn from the root canal. This action removes a portion of sealer out of the canal but leaves an adequate amount as a coating to the root canal walls.

## 2. Specially Designed Instruments used in a Reciprocating Handpiece

In order to overcome the danger of fracture inherent in rotating instruments the Giromatic* instrumentation was introduced in 1964. This consists of a right angled handpiece which accepts either specially designed barbed broaches or files and transforms the continuous rotation of the handpiece into an alternating quarter turn movement.

The advantages of this system over hand-operated instrumentation are that it allows good visibility thus making access into the canal openings easier. It is less arduous and, according to the manufacturer, five or six times quicker than conventional canal preparation. In those rare cases where rubber dam cannot be used it is, of course, safer because the broach is firmly attached to the handpiece.

The efficiency of the Giromatic system was compared with that of hand operated instruments by Harty and Stock (1974b) and Jungmann et al. (1975) who found that there was no difference between the systems and that neither system was adequate in preparing a canal to a round cross section in the apical fifth of the root.

However, there was no doubt that the Giromatic broaches were more flexible than the Giromatic Hedstroem-type files and these, in turn, more flexible than conventional Hedstroem files (Harty and Stock 1974a). This instrument flexibility, together with the safety factor, are the two chief advantages of the system.

The disadvantages are that tactile sense is lost but clinically this is not important because of the flexibility of the broaches and their blunt tips make perforation improbable. A more important disadvantage may be that the reciprocating action of the working point cuts dentine efficiently but makes its removal from the canal difficult. Ideally dentine chips should be removed as soon as they are detached from the canal walls lest they remain within the root canal and ultimately block it. This is particularly dangerous in teeth with fine canals. Thus if this system of instrumentation is to be used satisfactorily a period of mechanical cutting should be followed by rotary hand instrumentation so that the dentine debris may be removed.

---

*Micro-Mega S.A., 5–12 Rue du Tunnel, Besançon 25006, France.

Table 1.

| I.S.O. NUMBERS | 8 | 10 | 15 | 20 | 25 | 30 | 35 | 40 | 45 | 50 | 55 | 60 | 70 | 80 | 90 | 100 | 110 | 120 | 130 | 140 |
|---|---|---|---|---|---|---|---|---|---|---|---|---|---|---|---|---|---|---|---|---|
| Former M–M Numbers | 00 | 0 | 1 | 2 | 3 | 4 | | 5 | | 6 | | 7 | 8 | 9 | 10 | | | | | |
| Former Zipperer Numbers | 00 | | 1 | 2 | 3 | 4 | 5 | 6 | 7 | 8 | 9 | 10 | 11 | 12 | 13 | 14 | 15 | 16 | 17 | 18 |
| Giro-Broaches* | | | / | / | / | / | / | / | / | / | / | / | / | / | | | | | | |
| Giro-Files* | / | / | / | / | / | / | / | / | / | / | / | / | / | | | | | | | |
| Giro-Pointer* | | | / | / | / | / | / | / | | | | | | | | | | | | |
| Endomatic Barbed Broaches† | | | | | | / | / | / | / | / | / | / | / | / | | | | | | |
| Endomatic Plain Broaches† | | | / | / | / | / | / | / | / | / | / | / | / | / | | | | | | |

* Micro-Mega S.A., 5-12 Rue du Tunnel, Besançon 25006, France.
† Vereinigte Dentalwerke Antaeos-Beutelrock-Zipperer, Zdarsky Ehrler K.G., D 8 Munich 70, West Germany.

The instruments available for use with the Giromatic handpiece are given in *Table* 1 and are supplied in two lengths, 21 and 29 mm. The Giro-pointer is a short broach (16 mm) of one size only which facilitates the location of the canal and the enlargement of its orifice.

## V. AUXILIARY INSTRUMENTS

As in other fields of dentistry there is an abundance of subsidiary endodontic instruments which, their originators claim, must be used if a root filling is to be successful. A number of these are gimmicks which only work in the hands of their inventors. Others are useful in special situations.

### 1. *Safety Devices and the Rubber Dam*

Undoubtedly the use of the rubber dam (*see below*) gives the patient the best protection against the accidental inhalation or ingestion of instruments and drugs used in root therapy.

There are occasions when the use of the rubber dam is impossible, unnecessary or inconvenient. In such cases any instrument placed near the patient's mouth must be attached to a safety device which will make it impossible for the patient to swallow or inhale the instrument. Dental floss, black silk suture thread or specially manufactured chains can often be attached to the handle of the instrument, but these methods are seldom used because the preparation of each instrument is tedious and the extra bulk on the handle makes manipulation awkward.

To overcome these disadvantages Dimashkieh (1974) designed an instrument which holds reamers and files securely and allows them to be freely rotated within the canal and also has a variable angle of application.

### *Rubber Dam*

The use of the rubber dam, at least in the United Kingdom, is almost an emotional issue and some practitioners feel that it is an unnecessary, time consuming procedure. The question that must be asked is, 'Can one afford *not* to use it for root canal therapy, particularly if the patient is in the recumbent operating position?'

The purpose of the rubber dam is—

1. To protect the patient from the inhalation or ingestion of instruments, medicaments, tooth and filling debris and, possibly, bacteria and necrotic pulp tissue. The safety devices described previously are a substitute for the rubber dam and do not protect the patient fully.

2. To provide a clean dry sterilizable field of operation free from salivary contamination.

3. To prevent the tongue and cheeks from obstructing the operating field.

4. To prevent the patient from talking, washing out the mouth and generally interfering with the efficiency of the operator.

Rubber dam* is available in a variety of thicknesses (fine, medium, heavy and extra heavy) and colours (natural, grey, dark grey and black). It can be purchased in rolls or in pre-cut 5 or 6-inch squares. Choice of dam is, of course, a matter of personal preference, but for general all round use the dark grey or black heavy or extra heavy can be recommended because it has the advantage of a tight fit around the neck of the tooth thus providing a hermetic seal without the use of individual floss ligatures. It also has the advantage of not tearing easily and, because of its thickness, protects the underlying soft tissues effectively.

A number of frames are available and those that hold the dam away from the patient's face are preferred because they are more comfortable, cooler, drier and normally do not require an absorbent napkin between the dam and the patient's tissues. An example of such an instrument is the metal Fernald Ash rubber dam frame.† Plastic frames are also available and these have the advantage of being radiolucent (e.g. the Nygaard-Ostby frame‡ and the Starlite Visi-Frame§).

A rubber dam punch and a selection of clamps and clamp forceps are also necessary. Clamp selection need not be large and is a matter of individual preference. Ash Ivory's patterns† are useful because they have 'wings' which allow the clamp to be attached to the dam prior to tooth fixation (*Fig. 38*).

A basic assortment consists of the following:

Ash Ivory's Pattern 1 and 2A for bicuspids generally
6 and 9 for upper anterior teeth
7A and 27A for molars.

Dental floss, Orobase‖, wooden wedges and a flat plastic (No. 166) completes the kit.

As has been mentioned before, dental floss is generally not necessary as a ligature around the tooth but it is essential for testing the contacts between teeth prior to dam application. Orobase is often used on the tissue surface of the dam to facilitate placement and afford a better seal. Wooden wedges are useful in holding the

*Amalgamated Dental Co. Ltd., 26–40 Broadwick Street, London W1A 2AD or Hygienic Dental Manufacturing Co., Akron, Ohio, U.S.A. 44310.
†Amalgamated Dental Co. Ltd., 26–40 Broadwick St., London W1A 2AD.
‡Union Broach Co. Inc., 45–18 Court Square, Long Island N.Y. City, N.Y. 11101, U.S.A.
§Star Dental Mfg Co. Inc., Philadelphia, Pa. 19428, U.S.A.
‖E. R. Squibb & Sons Ltd., Regal House, Twickenham, Middlesex, U.K.

dam in place in cases where clamps cannot be used, for example where the tooth to be clamped has been restored with porcelain or bonded crown. The flat plastic instrument is useful in freeing the dam from the wings of the clamp and also in inverting and tucking in the dam in the gingival sulcus.

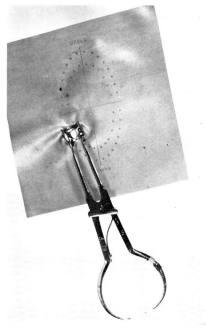

*Fig*. 38. Rubber dam attached to the 'wings' of an Ash Ivory pattern clamp.

## 2. *Measuring Stops, Gauges and Stands*

The importance of instrumentation to a known canal length has been stressed and there are several ways of marking instruments. They can be marked very simply by using marking paste (a mixture of petroleum jelly and zinc oxide) and an engineer's ruler. This method has the minor disadvantage that the paste can be wiped off easily and that there is no positive stop on the instrument.

Rubber stops, either specially manufactured or home made, provide an equally simple but more positive stop to instrumentation. A ruler is, of course, necessary to set the stops and various gadgets have been developed to make the setting operation easier. Rubber stops are difficult to use with the finer size of reamers and files because these instruments may be bent as they are pushed through the rubber (*Fig*. 39).

An improved metal stop and gauge* (*Fig.* 39a) has recently been devised and this has the advantage that the metal stop fits the shaft accurately and firmly and the stops are much smaller than conventional rubber stops.

Another ingenious system consists of clipping a plastic extension, of known length, into a groove in the handles of specially designed root therapy instruments† (*Fig.* 39c). In this way the working length of the instrument may be shortened and the handle extension provides the stop.

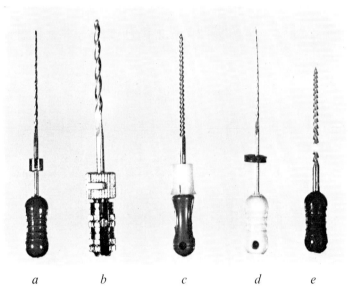

*a*          *b*          *c*          *d*          *e*

*Fig.* 39. Methods of marking instruments to the calculated canal length so that over-instrumentation can be avoided: *a*, Vari-Fix steel stop; *b*, Test handle system; *c*, Colorinox and Endomatic stop; *d*, Rubber stop; *e*, Marking paste.

The Test handle system‡ (*Fig.* 39b) consists of a handle, marked in millimetres, which accepts special reamers and files of various sizes. The handle can be tightened so that the working part is clamped at a predetermined length.

The advantage of the endomatic stop and the Test handle systems is that once fixed the stop will not slide even if force is applied. The disadvantages are expense and awkwardness in adjustment.

*Vari-Fix Steel Stop and Gauge: Vereinigte Dentalwerke Antaeos-Beutelrock-Zipperer, Zdarsky Ehrler K.G., D 8 Munich 70, West Germany.
†Colorinox and Endomatic Stops: Maillefer S.A., 1338 Ballaigues, Switzerland.
‡Vereinigte Dentalwerke Antaeos-Beutelrock-Zipperer, Zdarksy Ehrler K.G., D 8 Munich 70, West Germany.

To facilitate the accurate placement of rubber stops, various methods have been suggested (Guldener and Imobersteg, 1972; Rowe and Forrest, 1973) and one combines instrument measurement with a stand* (Barnard, 1974) (*Fig.* 40*a*).

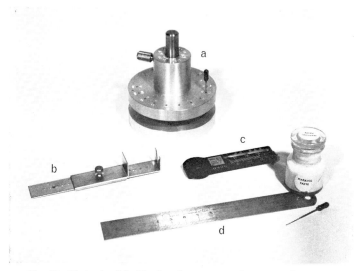

*Fig.* 40. Methods of facilitating the accurate placement of stops on the shaft of instruments: *a*, K.D. Endo. Gauge; *b*, Starlite measuring gauge; *c*, Vari-Fix gauge; *d*, Engineer's ruler and marking paste.

Stands are useful if instruments are to be placed in order and be easily accessible at the chairside. A number of these are commercially available (Endo-Magazine Endodontic Instrument Stand†, Davis Stand‡) but can also be home-made easily out of a length of aluminium angle (*Fig.* 41).

### 3. *Instruments for the Retrieval of Broken Instruments*

Prevention of this unfortunate accident is much easier than the removal of the fractured instrument from the root canal. This has been discussed in Chapter 11. The instruments used for the operation are fine beaked forceps and specially designed trephines.

Forceps can only be used if the end of the fractured instrument or silver point is visible and it is not jammed firmly within the canal.

---

*K.D. Endo. Gauge: K.R.D., Manchester M3 2AD, United Kingdom.

†'Endo-Magazine': Vereinigte Dentalwerke Antaeos-Beutelrock-Zipperer, Zdarsky Ehrler K.G., D 8 Munich 70, West Germany.

‡J. & S. Davis Ltd.: Cordent House, Torrington Park, London N12 9SX.

Fine beaked haemostats are sometimes useful, but grooved beaked forceps or Steiglitz ring-type forceps* will give a better chance of success.

If the instrument or point is jammed firmly it must be freed for part of its length so as to reduce the frictional resistance. This is a difficult operation which becomes relatively simple by using the Masserann (1971) technique and a specially manufactured kit.†

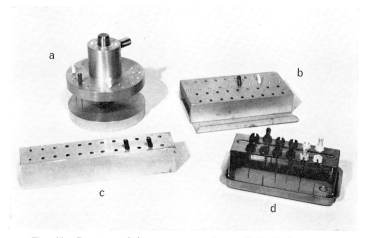

*Fig.* 41.   Root canal instrument stands: *a*, K.D. Endo. gauge; *b*, J. & S. Davis stand; *c*, Home-made stand; *d*, Endo-Magazine.

The principle of this method consists of freeing the broken fragment around its periphery and this is carried out by using a hollow trepan bur whose inner diameter corresponds to the diameter of the broken fragment. The advantage of this method is that the fragment itself acts as a guide and prevents the creation of a false pathway and possible perforation of the root. The 'trench' created around the broken instrument reduces the resistance of the fragment to removal and also creates space that allows the insertion of a second instrument which grips and extracts the broken fragment.

The kit is available in a box containing (*Fig.* 42)—

*a.* Fourteen colour-coded trepan burs which increase in diameter from 1·1 to 2·4 mm. The wall of the trepan is less than 0·25 mm.

*b.* Two handles which convert the trepan from a latch-type engine-operated instrument into one that can be hand-held.

---

*Star Dental Mfg Co. Inc., Philadelphia, Pa. 19428, U.S.A.
†Micro-Mega S.A., 5–12 Rue du Tunnel, Besançon 25006, France.

c. Two Masserann 'Star' gauges, each carrying seven tubes, the diameters of which progressively increase by 0·1 mm. These gauges facilitate the choice of trepan size.

d. A flat gauge which included a graduated tapered slot for checking the correct diameter of the trepan required for each case.

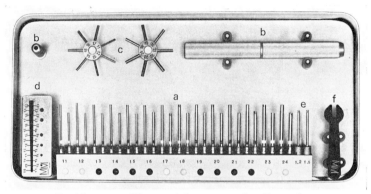

*Fig.* 42. Masserann Kit containing trepans, handles and gauges. (*Courtesy of Prodenta S.A., Micro-Mega Export.*)

e. Two Masserann extractors for use in the removal of fine broken root canal instruments, such as barbed broaches and fine reamers and files and also silver points.

f. A spanner for removing the trepans from the handles.

g. Two Gates drills (not shown).

*Method of Use*

a. *If the instrument is visible*, the diameter of the broken fragment is determined with the 'Star' gauge and a trench is cut around the fragment with the appropriate trepan. The fragment should be freed for about half its length.

Gripping and extraction of the fragment is carried out by using a trepan one size smaller than the one used to cut the trench around the broken instrument. By applying pressure, in an apical direction, the second trepan is friction fitted over the fractured instrument which can ultimately be rotated and removed.

This technique can be applied not only to broken endodontic instruments but also to posts that have fractured level with the tooth surface.

b. *If the fragment is not visible*, it is necessary to determine the diameter of the canal and this normally corresponds to the diameter of the broken invisible post or reamer. Because the diameter of the trepan to be used to remove the fractured instrument is greater than the canal diameter, it is necessary to enlarge it and this is done with a suitably sized trepan. This is, of course, a delicate operation and frequent radiographic check is necessary to make certain that the path being cut is in the correct plane.

When the fractured instrument is reached, a trench is cut around it and removed as described above.

Trepans should be used in slowly rotating handpieces or, preferably, by hand. They should be removed from the tooth frequently and the root irrigated, not only to wash out debris but also to cool the root which gets extremely hot even when the speed of trepanation is extremely slow.

*c. Fine instruments broken in the apical area.* The smallest trepan bur has a diameter of 1·1 mm and this is too large to engage a fine barbed broach or fine silver point. In these instances the use of the Masserann extractors is invaluable. These are supplied in two sizes and consist of a fine hollow tube which has an embossment on one end. The other end has a handle through which a stylet passes, and which, when fully seated, bears against the tube embossment. Fine fragments can be gripped by placing the tube over them and screwing the stylet until the fragment is secured against the internal embossment of the tube. Removal of the fractured fragment is then an easy matter.

The system has limitations and can only be used in straight canals or in canals which can be straightened. Nevertheless, the technique is to be commended for it simplifies and makes safe a relatively difficult operation.

### 4. *Instruments used in filling the Root Canal*

As has been mentioned previously, the object of any root canal filling procedure is the sealing of the canal contents from the peridental tissues. The instruments used to achieve this depend on the technique employed to obturate the canal.

*Single cone obturation.* No special instrumentation is required for this technique. Sealer is placed in the root canal with a spiral filler or with a reamer. The cone is lightly 'buttered' with sealer and placed at the correct level within the canal.

The usefulness of this technique is suspect and it has no advantage over other techniques except, possibly, simplicity.

Where this technique has to be used, e.g. in very fine canals of posterior teeth, then the empty spaces around the point in the middle and coronal third of the canal should be filled with a laterally condensed gutta percha root filling (*see below*). This is necessary because the incidence of lateral canals in the furcation areas of multi-rooted teeth is high and failure to obliterate this space may lead to periodontal problems.

*Sectional Techniques with Gutta Percha, Silver Points and Amalgam*
Specialized instrumentation is not required when using gutta percha or silver points (*see* Chapter 6).

However, when amalgam is the root filling of choice, then specially designed amalgam carriers and condensers are essential.

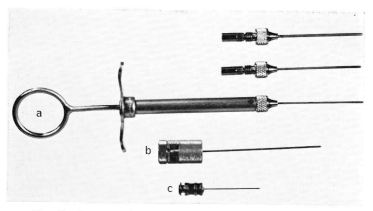

*Fig.* 43. Root canal therapy amalgam carriers: *a*, The 'P.D.' Messing root canal gun; *b*, Hill Endodontic amalgam carrier; *c*, Dimashkieh root canal amalgam carrier.

The three carriers (*Fig.* 43) described below are similar in design but vary in size. They are constructed of a tube with an accurately fitting plunger which allows small increments of amalgam to be picked up at the tip of the tube.

The amalgam is transferred to the root canal, and when the tube tip is at the correct level (and this can be checked radiographically) the amalgam is ejected from the tube by depressing the plunger. The amalgam is then condensed with a condenser made from a length of stainless-steel wire of suitable diameter.

The three commonly available carriers are:

*a. The 'P.D.' Messing Root Canal Gun\*:* This resembles a syringe and the plunger is spring loaded. It is supplied with three tube and plunger assemblies with outside diameters of 2·00, 1·50 and 1·00 mm. The larger diameters are too thick for conventional root fillings, but are useful for the retrograde filling of canals at apicectomy.

---

\*Produits Dentaires S.A., Vevey, Switzerland.

*b. The Hill Endodontic Amalgam Carrier\*:* This is a much smaller and simpler instrument without a spring loaded plunger and has an outside diameter of 0·90 mm. Both the above carriers have the following disadvantages. The shafts are not flexible and hence they can only be used in straight canals. Their overall size and relatively wide diameter confines their use to anterior teeth with large root canals.

*c. The Dimashkieh Root Canal Amalgam Carrier†:* This was designed specifically to overcome these problems and is, essentially, a much smaller version of the Hill carrier. It is available in three diameters (0·40, 0·50 and 0·60 mm) and each carrier is supplied with a matching condenser whose diameter is 0·05 mm less than the carrier. Both carriers and condensers are colour coded in the I.S.O. specification and are 31 mm in length. The shaft is flexible and because of its small overall length it is possible to use the instrument in posterior teeth which have relatively fine canals.

The instrument is, of course, delicate and must be used with care. On no account should the carrier be used as a condensing point lest the tip be damaged. Special stainless-steel wire condensers are provided. With these limitations, the author has found this carrier eminently suitable for sectional amalgam root filling. These instruments have been fully described by Messing (1958), Hill (1967) and Dimashkieh (1975).

*Lateral and Vertical Gutta Percha Condensation Techniques*

The instruments used in these techniques are not identical. Condensers are available as spreaders or pluggers. Both instruments have a tapered working point of about 30 mm. However, the ends of spreaders are pointed whilst pluggers have blunt ends. The former instruments are designed to condense gutta percha laterally against the walls of the root canal whilst pluggers have the dual function of condensing laterally and also vertically.

Generally, in the lateral condensation technique, spreaders are used cold and rely on pressure alone to condense gutta percha. This does not result in a root filling with a homogeneous mass of gutta percha but rather in one consisting of a series of separate points stuck together with sealer.

Schilder's vertical condensation technique utilizes considerable heat to soften the gutta percha points. This is achieved by the use of a spreader or 'heat carrier'. The softened gutta percha mass is then mechanically condensed with a cold plugger, which has been

---

*Percy J. Clark & Co. Ltd., Kemdent Works, Purton, Swindon, Wiltshire, U.K.
†Weshill Development Co., 26A Cleaver Square, Kennington, London S.E.11.

'dusted' with a dry zinc oxide powder to prevent adhesion of the warm gutta percha onto the plugger. Both spreaders and pluggers (*Fig.* 44) are generally available mounted on long handles so that control is easier and, the contra-angle variety can be used in posterior teeth. Luks has designed a series of four short finger pluggers* (really spreaders, for they all have sharp points) which are mounted on handles similar to reamers. The short length of these instruments affords a higher degree of tactile sense and allows the instruments to be rotated freely around their axes in both directions, thus freeing the instrument for easy removal (*Fig.* 44*d*).

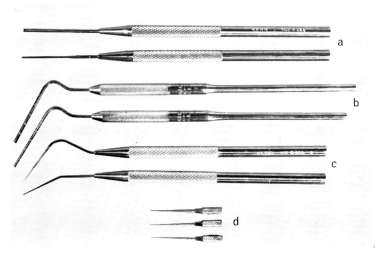

*Fig.* 44. Instruments used in lateral and vertical condensation techniques: *a*, Condensers for use in anterior teeth; *b*, Condensers for use in posterior teeth; *c*, Spreaders; *d*, Luks short finger pluggers.

## VI. STORAGE AND STERILIZATION OF INSTRUMENTS

Whilst it is generally recognized that sterility within the root canal can never be achieved, instruments used in the root canal must be sterile and not just surgically clean or disinfected.

Prearranged sets of instruments can be sterilized and stored in metal boxes. These are available in a variety of sizes with or without compartments. Some have been specially designed to take a full complement of endodontic instrumentation. One such box is the

*Starlite Stainless Finger Pluggers: Star Dental Mfg Co. Inc., Philadelphia, Pa. 19428, U.S.A.

RAF model* which has a stand for reamers and files, a 'clean grip' for cleaning reamers, medicament trays, pellet containers, etc. (*Fig.* 45).

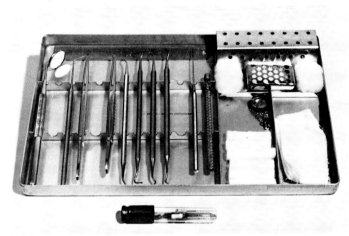

*Fig.* 45. Metal box (R.A.F. model) designed to hold a full complement of endodontic instrumentation. Note that reamers and files are sterilized and stored in test tubes and not in the metal box.

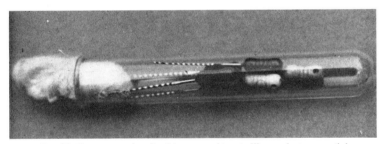

*Fig.* 46. Pyrex test tubes 3 × ½ in are used to sterilize and store partial sets of root canal hand instruments.

Complete sets of reamers, files, fillers, etc. should never be included in the basic instrumentation boxes, for one seldom uses more than one length of instrument in any particular tooth. A better method may be to store a portion of a set, say No. 15–40 of 25 mm length in 3 by ½ in Pyrex test tubes (*Fig.* 46). In this way only the test tube containing the set that is going to be used is opened and there is no need to re-sterilize the entire set with consequent deterioration of the physical properties of each instrument.

*J. & S. Davis Ltd., Cordent House, Torrington Park, London N12 9SX.

89

These test tubes can also be used to store, and keep sterile, sets of other small instruments, such as spiral fillers, burs and paper points. The latter are also available in pre-sterilized packs in one of the five different sizes*

### Sterilization of Endodontic Instruments

Various methods are advocated and these are: (1) Chemical disinfection; (2) Boiling water disinfection; (3) Dry heat sterilization; (4) Bead, salt or molten metal sterilization; (5) Pressure steam (autoclaving) sterilization; (6) 'Gas' sterilization.

### 1. Chemical 'Disinfectants' or 'Cold' Sterilizers

These are in common use but have no place in endodontic practice because their disinfecting properties are inhibited by serum and other organic materials. Their action is selective and their effect on spores and viruses is often poor and unpredictable. Chemicals may cause metal instruments to rust and cannot be used for the disinfection of cotton materials and paper points.

### 2. Boiling Water Disinfection

Water at normal atmosphere and pressure boils at 100° C. This temperature is not sufficient to destroy spores and, indeed, it will not destroy viruses if protected by serum or other organic matter. Again this method is not recommended for endodontic instruments. Certain materials, such as paper points, cannot be sterilized by this method.

### 3. Dry Heat Sterilization

This is the method of choice because it is effective on all endodontic instruments. Both hand instruments and other materials, such as cottonwool and paper points, can be placed in one box, sterilized, and sealed where they remain sterile for an indefinite period. The disadvantage of this method lies in the fact that relatively high temperatures are required if the sterilization time is to be reasonably short and this may affect the finish and temper of instruments repeatedly sterilized.

The recommended dry heat sterilization temperature is 160° C for 45 minutes. This is chosen because cottonwool and paper points char at higher temperatures. Thus with the preheating time and the cooling down period after sterilization, the total time required for the cycle is about 90 minutes.

Inexpensive dry heat sterilizers are readily available. However, if such a sterilizer is not available, sterilization can be carried out in an ordinary domestic oven. A gas oven can be set at Regulo 3,

---

*Johnson & Johnson Ltd., 260 Bath Road, Slough, Bucks SL1 4EA.

which gives a temperature of 163° C (325° F). Modern electric ovens may be more suitable, because temperature control is more accurate and heat distribution is more effective due to the incorporation of a fan which circulates the hot air.

The efficiency of hot air sterilization can be checked by using Browne's Tubes (type 3)*, the colour of which alters from red to green once the correct temperature and time have been reached. A tube should be placed in the middle of the batch of instruments to be sterilized so that the check is made on the most inaccessible area of the package.

Dry heat sterilization indicator tapes† are heat sensitive and the stripes on the tape turn from pale green to brown upon exposure to dry heat at 160° C. They are used to differentiate items that have been processed by dry heat from those that have not and they should never be used as providing proof of sterility.

### 4. *Bead, Salt or Molten Metal Sterilization*
These methods are effective provided the instrument to be sterilized is held in the heat conducting material for a minimum of 10 seconds. Strict adherence to this rule makes the process very time consuming. Metal and bead sterilizers have also been criticized because it is relatively easy to carry metal fragments or beads into the root canals and cause an obstruction. Further, variation in temperature within the well are common and may lead to imperfect sterilization. These sterilizers are normally electrically operated but Johns (1970) has described a gas operated model.

### 5. *Pressure Steam (Autoclaving) Sterilization*
This is effective and has the advantage of a reasonably short cycle—three minutes at 134° C. However, for effective sterilization to take place all air must be removed from the sterilizing chamber and, ideally, a vacuum should be established. This makes even the simplest machines expensive. Other disadvantages are that cotton-wool and paper points have to be dried after sterilization and non-stainless-steel endodontic instruments may rust.

### 6. *'Gas' Sterilization*
Sterilizers using ethylene oxide, alcohol and other chemicals are available, and these have the advantage of operating at lower temperatures reached much quicker than conventional water autoclaves. Because water is not present in the system, cotton wool and paper points are dry and ready for use as soon as the cycle is complete.

---

*Albert Browne Ltd., Chancery House, Abbey Gate, Leicester LE4 0AA.
†Indair Dry Heat Sterilisation Indicator Tape. No. 1226: 3M United Kingdom Ltd., 3M House, Wigmore Street, London W1A 1ET.

## VII. STANDARDIZED INSTRUMENTS

Until fairly recently root canal hand instruments and filling points were not standardized in size, shape or length and each manufacturer numbered his range of instruments differently. Moreover there was only accidental agreement between the size of instruments and filling points used to obturate the canal (Green, 1957).

The use of instruments whose taper varied from one number to the next sometimes led to fracture of the instrument because the tip 2 or 3 mm could jam against the canal walls (*Fig.* 47).

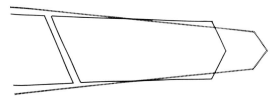

*Fig.* 47. The dotted line represents a root canal prepared with an instrument of a certain taper. If an attempt is now made to enlarge this canal with an instrument of different taper the tip is likely to jam and the instrument may fracture.

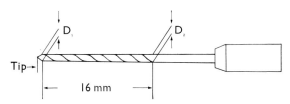

*Fig.* 48. Diagrammatic representation of reamer and file. Note that $D_2 = D_1 + 0.32$ mm and that the taper proportion is $0.02 : 1$ mm.

Ingle (1955, 1956) and others saw the need for standardization as early as 1955 and their proposals were placed before the Second International Conference on Endodontics (1958), which accepted the following:

1. A formula for the diameter and taper of each instrument and filling point.

2. A formula for the graduated increase in size from one instrument to the next.

3. A new instrument-numbering system based on the diameter of the instrument.

The standardization was accomplished by the following method (*Fig.* 48):

1. Diameter 1 ($D_1$) was measured in millimetres, at a point the instrument blades begin at the tip of the instrument.

2. Diameter 2 ($D_2$) was a point at which the working blades terminated and which was 16 mm from point $D_1$. Further, point $D_2$ was to be 0·3 mm greater in diameter than $D_1$.

Thus by standardizing the length of the cutting blade and also the increase in diameter from $D_1$ to $D_2$ the taper from one instrument to the next was uniform and depended on the following formulae:

$$\frac{D_2 - D_1}{\text{Length between } D_2 \text{ and } D_1} = \frac{0·3 \text{ mm}}{16·0 \text{ mm}}$$

$$= 0·01874 \text{ increase per mm of blade.}$$

3. The instruments were numbered according to the diameter $D_1$ and the number was stated as the diameter at $D_1$ in millimetres $\times 100$. E.g., If the diameter at $D_1$ were 0·45 mm the number given on the instrument was 45.

4. The progressive increase in size from one instrument to the next was to be 0·05 mm (50 microns) up to a No. 60 and 0·1 mm (100 microns) thereafter.

5. Silver points were to be given the same number as the corresponding reamers and files but their diameter at any point was to be 0·009 mm (9 microns) smaller, so as to compensate for the thickness of the cementing medium and the dentine compressibility during instrumentation.

6. Tolerances allowed for reamers and files at $D_1$ and $D_2$ were $\pm 0·00$ mm and $+0·00$ mm and $-0·01$ mm for silver points.

The matter has been considered by the International Standards Organization who have published the following Draft Specifications which uses a coding directly related to the significant dimensions of the instrument. It must be emphasized that this is a Draft which has not, as yet, been ratified (International Standards Organization, 1975).

The draft specifies the dimensions, the designations and a system of colour coding for hand- and motor-operated reamers and files designed for the mechanical reshaping and surface preparation of root canals.

The diameters $D_1$ and $D_2$ of the operative end (illustrated in *Fig.* 48) shall correspond to those detailed in *Table* 2 for the relevant nominal size designation.

The number given to the instrument is the tip diameter in hundredths of a millimetre, i.e. if the diameter at $D_1$ is 0·45 mm the number given to the instrument will be 0·45 × 100 = 45.

The length of the operative end shall be one of the following: 21, 25, 28, 31 mm with a tolerance, in each instance, of $\pm 0·5$ mm.

The taper of the operative end shall be 1 : 50, i.e. an increase of 0·02 millimetres per 1·00 millimetre.

The tip length for twisted instruments, excepting the Hedstroem file, shall not exceed the diameter $D_1$, or 1 mm, whichever is the lesser. The tip length of the Hedstroem file shall not be greater than twice $D_1$. (Thus Hedstroem files may have longer and much sharper tips than other instruments.)

The colour coding suggested is given in *Table* 2.

*Table* 2.

| Colour Coding | Nominal Size Designation | Diameter $D_1$ ($\pm 0{\cdot}02$ mm) | Diameter $D_2$ ($\pm 0{\cdot}02$ mm) |
|---|---|---|---|
| | | mm | mm |
| Purple | 010 | 0·10 | 0·42 |
| White | 015 | 0·15 | 0·47 |
| Yellow | 020 | 0·20 | 0·52 |
| Red | 025 | 0·25 | 0·57 |
| Blue | 030 | 0·30 | 0·62 |
| Green | 035 | 0·35 | 0·67 |
| Black | 040 | 0·40 | 0·72 |
| White | 045 | 0·45 | 0·77 |
| Yellow | 050 | 0·50 | 0·82 |
| Red | 055 | 0·55 | 0·87 |
| Blue | 060 | 0·60 | 0·92 |
| Green | 070 | 0·70 | 1·02 |
| Black | 080 | 0·80 | 1·12 |
| White | 090 | 0·90 | 1·22 |
| Yellow | 100 | 1·00 | 1·32 |
| Red | 110 | 1·10 | 1·42 |
| Blue | 120 | 1·20 | 1·52 |
| Green | 130 | 1·30 | 1·62 |
| Black | 140 | 1·40 | 1·72 |

Whilst the specifications given above have not been ratified most manufacturers have already accepted the I.S.O. recommendations and use these to produce instruments labelled 'Standardized' or 'ISO Sizes'.

REFERENCES

Barnard D. (1974) The carousel endometer. *J. Br. Endodont. Soc.* **7**, 28.

Dimashkieh M. R. (1974) Applicator for root canal instruments. *Br. Dent. J.* **137**, 359.

Dimashkieh M. R. (1975) A method of using silver amalgam in routine endodontics, and its use in open apices. *Br. Dent. J.* **138**, 298.

Fauchard P. (1746) *The Surgeon Dentist*, trans. from 2nd ed. by L. Lindsay. London, Butterworths, 1946.

Green E. N. (1957) Microscopic investigation of root canal file and reamer widths. *Oral Surg.* **10**, 532.

Guldener P. H. and Imobersteg C. (1972) New method of measuring the exact length of root canal instruments. *J. Br. Endodont. Soc.* **6**, 51.

Harty F. J. and Sondoozi A. E. (1972) The status of standardised endodontic instruments. *J. Br. Endodont. Soc.* **6**, 57.

Harty F. J. and Stock C. J. R. (1974a) A comparison of the flexibility of giromatic and hand operated instruments in endodontics. *J. Br. Endodont. Soc.* **7**, 64.

Harty F. J. and Stock C. J. R. (1974b) The giromatic system compared with hand instrumentation in endodontics. *Br. Dent. J.* **137**, 239.

Hill T. R. (1967) An amalgam carrier for use in endodontic treatment. *Dent. Pract. Dent. Rec.* **17**, 285.

Ingle J. I. (1955) The need for endodontic instrument standardization. *Oral Surg.* **8**, 1211.

Ingle J. I. (1956) Root canal obturation. *J. Am. Dent. Assoc.* **53**, 47.

Ingle J. I. and Le Vine M. (1958) In: Grossman L. I. (ed.), *Transactions of the Second International Conference on Endodontics.* Philadelphia, University of Pennsylvania, p. 123.

International Standards Organization (1975) *Dental Root Canal Reamers and Files—Part I: Nominal Size, Dimensions and Colour Coding.* DIS 3630.

Johns R. B. (1970) A small steriliser for endodontic instruments. *J. Br. Endodont. Soc.* **4**, 12.

Jungmann C. L., Uchin R. A. and Butcher J. F. (1975) Effect of instrumentation of the shape of the root canal. *J. Endodont.* **1**, 66.

Luks S. (1959) An analysis of root canal instruments. *J. Am. Dent. Assoc.* **58**, 85.

Masserann J. (1971) Translation of: *Entfern metallischer Fragmente aus Wurzelkanalen. J. Br. Endodont. Soc.* **5**, 55.

Messing J. J. (1958) Obliteration of the apical third of the root canal with amalgam. *Br. Dent. J.* **104**, 125.

Rowe A. H. R. and Forrest J. O. (1973) The endo-meter: A new method for adjusting the length of root canal instruments. *Br. Dent. J.* **134**, 437.

Tidmarsh B. G. (1975) Endodontic spiral root fillers. *J. Endodont. Soc.* **8**, 104.

# CHAPTER 6

# CONVENTIONAL ROOT CANAL THERAPY I
## The Preparation and Medication of the Root Canal

ROOT CANAL therapy can be defined as the treatment of the non-vital tooth, or of the dying tooth, of which the pulp is so badly injured that it must be removed completely and the root canal treated if the tooth is to be kept in function. It also includes cases where the pulp has to be removed electively because the canal has to be used in a post-retained restoration.

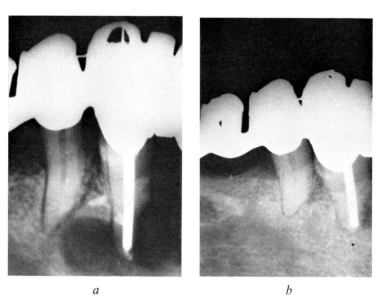

*a*                                    *b*

*Fig.* 49. The size of the area is not a criterion for surgery. *a*, Radiograph on completion of conventional root filling showing large cyst-like area of rarefaction and apical resorption. *b*, Radiograph 15 months later showing nearly complete bone healing.

This treatment may be carried out either by *conventional means*, i.e. through an access cavity in the crown of the tooth, or by *surgical means*. In both cases the aim of the treatment is to seal the canal contents from the periapical tissues.

The rationale of treatment relies on the fact that normal periapical tissues can well resist infection, but the dead pulp of a tooth, being avascular, has no defence mechanisms and forms an excellent, warm, moist culture medium. Even in the absence of bacterial invasion, autolysis of pulp tissue takes place and irritant or toxic breakdown products diffuse into the surrounding tissues. Furthermore, it is not enough to empty the canal, as it will rapidly fill with a seepage of tissue fluid and this, in turn, breaks down, diffuses into the periapical area and causes periapical irritation. Therefore, apart from the

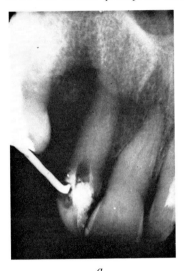 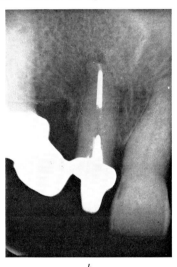

a            b

*Fig.* 50. *a,* Non-vital 2| with considerable distal bone loss simulating a combined endodontic/periodontic lesion. *b,* Radiograph 12 months later showing bone deposition following conventional root canal therapy using a sectional silver point technique. The lesion was obviously of endodontic origin.

necessity of removing the source of infection and the cleaning of the canal both mechanically and by irrigation, the apical 3 mm must ultimately be sealed so that neither bacteria nor toxic products can reach the periapical tissues, nor tissue fluids seep in.

Before a decision is made on the method to be used in dealing with the case, the patient must be treated for the relief of pain, and this has been discussed in Chapter 11.

## CHOICE OF CONSERVATIVE OR SURGICAL TREATMENT

Neither the size of the area of rarefaction nor the severity of any acute abscess nor the presence of chronic infection draining through a sinus are definite indications for surgery. Even an area of rarefaction as large as 1 cm in diameter is rarely cystic (*Figs.* 49, 50).

All cases may be treated conservatively in the first instance except—

1. Where it is not possible to cleanse the canal and seal the apex, e.g.:
   i.   An open apical foramen.
   ii.  A sharp bend in the apical third of the root canal.
   iii. An immovable obstruction in the canal.
   iv.  More than one apical foramen to the canal.
   v.   Where an adequate restoration exists (e.g. a porcelain jacket crown) and which is electively not disturbed. Generally it is possible to obtain access into the pulp chamber by boring through the crown. There is a risk of crown fracture but this does not usually occur unless an instrument is twisted against the walls of the access cavity.
2. Where the patient has not the time for a course of conservative treatment.
3. Where antibiotic cover is needed for each session of the treatment, e.g. in patients with rheumatic heart disease.

## METHOD AND RATIONALE

It is assumed that the tooth to be treated has always been symptomless or has become so following the emergency treatment described in Chapter 11.

### Isolation and Disinfection of the Crown

It is evident that steps must be taken to avoid infecting an uninfected tooth, and, when dealing with an infected canal, to reduce the introduction of further organisms to an absolute minimum. This involves: (1) The preparation and isolation of the clinical crown; (2) The disinfection of the crown and its immediate environment; (3) The use of a surgically clean technique.

### 1. The Preparation of the Crown

The preparation of the crown necessitates the removal of all caries, and the filling (temporary or permanent) of axial cavities, preferably with amalgam. Isolation is achieved by means of rubber dam which is easily placed and convenient to use. The patient cannot close his mouth or chatter, instruments cannot drop into the mouth or throat, and unpleasant medicaments do not reach the patient. This is all in addition to the main purpose of the technique which is that salivary seepage into the tooth is eliminated and bacterial contamination therefore largely avoided. The dam is placed most easily on upper anterior teeth and the beginner should start with these. Holes are punched into the dam in the form of the arch having first marked these points with a pencil on the dam over the teeth; then the rubber is placed over the teeth and held with rubber dam clamps.

A clamp placed on the tooth being operated on may hinder the position of the radiograph. Clamps placed further back in the mouth will hold the rubber away from the tooth concerned, and so allow easier manipulation of instruments and the placing of the radiograph. A rubber dam may be positioned on posterior teeth by first slipping the rubber over the special wings of the clamp, applying the clamp to the tooth and then releasing the rubber to position itself around the neck of the tooth (*Fig.* 38). The frame is then placed on the dam to hold it away from the patient's face. The instrumentation required for rubber dam placement has been described in Chapter 5.

If it is not possible to isolate the tooth and protect the patient's oro-pharynx with a rubber dam then other precautions must be taken to prevent saliva seeping into the root canals and particularly the accidental swallowing or inhalation of the delicate root therapy instruments and medicaments. The tooth may be isolated by means of cottonwool rolls or gauze squares, which can be conveniently kept in position by the use of a rubber dam clamp alone. Useful and absorbent cheek guards* are also available.

If a rubber dam is not used all hand-held root canal instruments should be attached to a safety device (*Fig.* 51).

In posterior teeth, where access is difficult, the instruments may be held in Spencer-Wells artery forceps, and instrumentation carried out by a filing rather than a reaming action. The Micro-Mega Giromatic handpiece† has been described on p. 76 and has much to commend it because the enlarging barbed broach or file is held firmly in the handpiece.

Some manufacturers produce long-handled files and reamers (*Fig.* 51*a*) and these ensure that the instrument will not be swallowed accidentally even if dropped in the mouth. A suitably trimmed anaesthetic throat pack or a folded gauze square is a further pre-caution against swallowed instruments.

If, in spite of all the precautions taken, an instrument is lost the practitioner must arrange immediate X-rays of both the chest and abdomen so that its precise location can be ascertained. If the instrument is in the abdomen its passage through the alimentary canal must be checked daily until, as normally happens, it is excreted. A much more serious situation exists if the instrument is not excreted or is inhaled, when surgical intervention is usually inevitable.

---

*'Dry guards' Virilium Co. Ltd., 46–48 Pentonville Road, London N1.
†Micro-Mega S.A., 5–12 Rue du Tunnel, Besançon 25006, France.

In either case the practitioner must inform his Medical Protection Society at once, because litigation is almost certain to follow such an unfortunate and easily preventable accident.

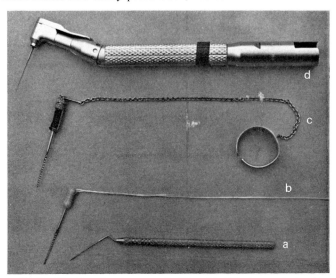

*Fig.* 51. If rubber dam is not used all hand-held instruments should be attached to a safety device. For example: *a*, File mounted on long hangle; *b*, Floss or black silk attached to reamer handle; *c*, Specially designed safety chain; *d*, The use of Micro-Mega instrumentation. It must be emphasized that these are inadequate and cumbersome substitutes for the rubber dam.

## 2. *The Disinfection of the Crown*

The rubber dam is placed on the appropriate teeth and the crowns and dam surrounding them are disinfected by swabbing with a 5 per cent solution of Savlon (I.C.I.) which contains chlorhexidine (Hibitane) 1·5 per cent w/v+cetrimide (Cetavlon) 15 per cent w/v. Seventy per cent iso-propyl alcohol may be used but is less effective and iodine may stain the tooth unnecessarily. Either Hibitane or Cetavlon used alone are reasonably effective.

## 3. *Surgical Cleanliness*

The total number of organisms that enter the field must be kept to a minimum and no pathogens should be introduced. All instruments must be sterilized at the beginning of the operation (*see* Chapter 5) and must not thereafter be contaminated except by the contents of the canal in question. If two teeth are being treated at the same time a different set of instruments must be used for each unless their areas of pathology are in continuity apically, as their bacterial flora may not be identical.

*Access*

It is now necessary to gain adequate access to the pulp cavity. A carious cavity leading into the canal is often present, but this is seldom the access of choice. Usually this should be filled (it *must* be excavated and rendered caries free) and a new access cavity made.

The guiding principles in designing such a cavity are:

i.   Its shape must be such that instruments are not deflected by the access cavity walls as these are passed to the apex of the root canal(s).

ii.  It must be large enough to allow complete débridement of the pulp chamber. Too small a cavity allows infected material to be retained within the pulp chamber and this may be transferred inadvertently to the root canal during subsequent instrumentation.

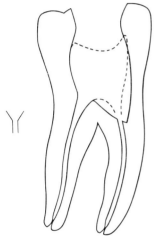

Fig. 52. The floor of the pulp chamber above the mesial canal has been over-instrumented, thus destroying the smooth funnel-shaped orifice into the canal and also reducing its diameter.

iii. The cavity must not be excessively large because this may seriously weaken the tooth. It is said that the dentine of root filled teeth is more brittle than that of vital teeth. Renson (1971) has shown that this is not so, and the fact that root filled teeth fracture more readily than vital teeth is due to the weakening of the crown by the access cavity and of the root by the enlargement of the canal during instrumentation.

iv.  The floor of the pulp chamber of posterior teeth must not be disturbed because the orifices of root canals are usually funnel-shaped and removal of tissues in the area reduces the diameter of the conical opening which makes subsequent instrumentation more difficult (*Fig.* 52).

To follow these principles a knowledge of pulpal anatomy is essential (*see* Chapter 3).

## Method

Access into the pulp chamber should be a two-stage operation. An ultra-high-speed instrument is used for the initial penetration through enamel and the cavity extended to form the correct outline. This preparation should normally be carried out prior to the placement of a rubber dam, which may obscure the root angulation and other anatomical features, and this, in turn, may lead to the perforation of the root during instrumentation (*Fig.* 53). On completion of the first stage the rubber dam may be placed, and the area cleansed and disinfected.

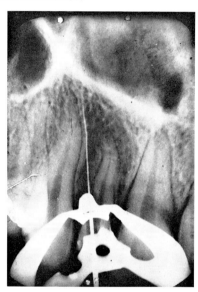

*Fig.* 53. Eccentric placement of rubber dam clamp has led to the masking of the root angulation and other anatomical features and this, in turn, has resulted in root perforation.

The second stage is carried out with conventional speed handpieces utilizing round or pear-shaped burs only. Bearing in mind the anatomy and direction of the pulp chamber the roof is penetrated and removed using a 'pull stroke'. Care is taken not to damage the walls and, more importantly, the floor of the pulp chamber. An aspirator is useful as it prevents debris from dropping into the canals of the teeth.

### Removal of Tissue

Local analgesia is necessary only if there is vital tissue in the tooth.

#### 1. *Vital Teeth*

In teeth with a single straight canal the pulp chamber contents and radicular pulp are removed together using barbed broaches. A single broach of correct size is sufficient for a narrow canal, but if this is of large cross section then two or three broaches are inserted together. The broaches should not be allowed to bind against the walls of the canal nor reach the apical foramen. They should be inserted into the pulp tissue, rotated through an angle of 90°, so that the barbs engage, and removed. Over-zealous rotation of the barbed broach(es) should be avoided as it may lead to tissue fragmentation and incomplete pulp removal.

If the pulp is not removed in one piece a second attempt with a new broach will be necessary. Broaches are difficult to clean at the chairside and should be discarded after a single use.

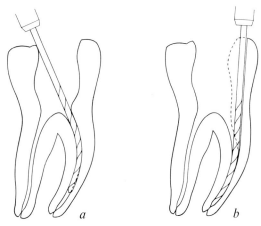

*Fig.* 54. *a*, Because of curve in mesial root canal the instrument has to be bent excessively. Instrumentation is difficult and may lead to ledge formation and/or perforation. *b*, Removal of tissue from the mesial wall of the access cavity and the root canal allows instrumentation to proceed without undue bending of the file.

In multi-rooted teeth pulp removal should be a two-stage operation. Firstly, pulp chamber contents are removed with sharp long shaft excavators (e.g. Ash No. 139/140 or No. 125/126) so that the openings of the root canals are visible. Secondly, each radicular pulp is extirpated by using barbed broaches as described above. Very fine canals can not be instrumented with barbed broaches because of their relatively large diameter. In these cases fine Hedstroem or rat-tail files are useful.

### 2. *Non-vital Teeth*

The débridement of non-vital teeth is more difficult, and both barbed broaches and files may be used. The instrument is inserted into the canal for about 3 mm and the canal contents engaged by rotating the instrument through an angle of 90°. The instrument is then removed, and in the case of files cleansed on a sterile napkin, cottonwool roll or rubber dam, and then re-inserted to engage a further portion of pulpal tissue. The canal is thus cleaned in stages.

In curved canals, débridement and canal exploration are carried out with a fine file of which the tip 3 mm has been held in a sterile napkin and bent, with the fingers, into a gentle curve. The direction of the curve should be marked on the instrument handle so that the tip of the instrument may be directed along the curvature of the canal. Insertion, removal and cleaning are carried out as before. Where the canal is found to be very curved, the occlusal portion of the canal may have to be enlarged and the canal 'straightened' by filing (*not* reaming) until the exploring file can be passed approximately to the apex (*Fig.* 54).

Mechanical instrumentation, e.g. by the Micro-Mega Giromatic handpiece, is considered by some to be an aid in the initial penetration of fine root canals (*see* p. 76).

### *Measurement of Canal Length*

It is now necessary to accurately know the length of the canal. A reamer or file of which the shaft is slightly longer than the tooth and of which the tip is about the same diameter as the apical portion of the root canal (as determined from the preoperative radiograph and average tooth lengths) is passed gently up the root canal until the instrument is impeded by the apical constriction. This is usually 0·5–1 mm from the apical foramen. The instrument is marked at a point level with a landmark such as the incisal edge, and a radiograph is taken (instrument stops are discussed on p. 80). It is then withdrawn and the length from its tip to the mark is measured and recorded.

When the X-ray is developed the procedure is repeated, if necessary, until the instrument is within 1 mm of the radiographic apex. The length of the tooth is now known accurately. All subsequent instrumentation is carried out to within 0·5–1 mm of the apex, and within this millimetre errors due to bending of the film and angulation of the X-ray beam are likely to be slight. The use of the formula—

$$\text{Canal length} = \frac{\text{Radiographic length of tooth} \times \text{actual length of instrument}}{\text{Radiographic length of instrument}}$$

for the calculation of the length of the root canal may lead to error due to the bending of the film in the mouth and also because it is difficult to measure accurately the radiographic length of tooth and instrument.

It is worth recalling that canals do not necessarily end at the anatomical or radiographic apex of the root: in fact more frequently they open to one side and the apical foramen is about 0·5–1 mm short of the anatomical apex. This is probably the ideal length to aim at and most surveys have shown that teeth filled just short of the radiographic apex are more often successful than those filled flush or over-filled (Seltzer et al., 1963; Ingle, 1965; Harty et al., 1970).

### Cleansing the Canal

The importance of removing debris and infected dentine as early as possible cannot be over-emphasized. The correct instrumentation, debridement and root filling of the canal, without the use of any sterilizing agent, can often lead to a successful result. The converse,

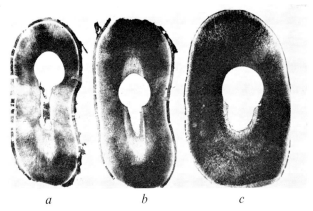

| *a* | *b* | *c* |

*Fig.* 55. Instrumentation of ribbon-shaped canal. *a*, Initial penetration with reamer produces near-round preparation along a section of the canal. *b* and *c*, Adequate débridement can only be completed by filing.

is not true. No amount of chemotherapy, unless preceded by correct and adequate instrumentation, will lead to a satisfactory result. This fact, therefore, places in a suspect category any endodontic techniques that advocate the use of medicaments without mechanical cleaning of the root canal. Softened dentine, which in any case is heavily contaminated, must be removed from the walls of the canal so that a seal can be established between the filling material and sound dentine.

Reamers and files are used for this part of the treatment. Reamers open up the canal and shape the apical portion, while files reach the elliptical areas not accessible to reamers (*Fig.* 55). These instruments should be used by hand and even so it is easy enough to perforate the root or break an instrument. Engine reamers magnify these possibilities and have no place in safe root canal therapy.

Controversy exists about the relative merits of the use of reamers and files. Some operators feel that reamers should be used exclusively whilst others counsel the reverse. In fact what is important is the method of use. Both reamers and files used *with a reaming action*, in a straight canal where the instrument is not bent, produce nearly round clinically acceptable preparations. Files, on the other hand when used *with a filing action* produce significant deviations from preparations that are uniformly circular in cross-section (Vessey, 1968; Harty and Stock, 1974; Jungmann et al., 1975).

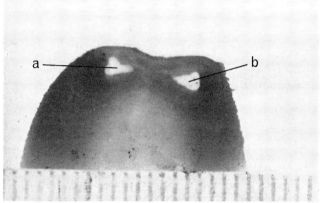

*Fig.* 56. Mesial root of first mandibular molar sectioned 3 mm from apex. *a*, Mesiobuccal canal had been mechanically instrumented with Giro file. *b*, Mesiolingual canal instrumented with hand-held Hedstroem file. Note that both preparations are irregular in cross section and not circular as expected. (*Photograph by courtesy of Major C. J. R. Stock.*)

Besides the removal of infected dentine the object of canal instrumentation is to prepare the apical 4–5 mm to such a size, cross-section and taper, that the obturating point will fit the prepared cavity perfectly. This implies that the cross-section must be circular and thus this area should be prepared with either files or reamers *used with a reaming action only*. Ribbon-shaped or widely flaring canals coronal to the apical area should be prepared with files used with a filing action.

In the case of curved canals, irrespective of the method of use, and the instrument used, the apical 4–5 mm of prepared canal will be oval in cross section (Harty and Stock, 1974). This is so because files and reamers are not sufficiently flexible, and tend to cut an eccentric cavity as they are manipulated (*Fig.* 56).

With these limitations in mind the canal is enlarged until all infected dentine is removed and irregularities in the canal walls smoothed out. The following method is suggested:

1. Ream to within 0·5–1 mm of the radiographic apex of the tooth until clean white dentine is cut by the reamer.

2. Use reamer and file sizes consecutively and in progression up the scale so that step formation is avoided.

3. Try to avoid forcing debris through the apex by constant withdrawal and wiping of the instrument on a sterile cotton-wool roll: the instrument should only be given half a turn before each withdrawal to enable the filings which cling to the instrument to be removed with it. A test with an extracted tooth is instructive and shows just how easy it is to push material through the apex.

4. Avoid bending reamers more than 30°. It is usually not possible to bend reamers or files even to this angle if the diameter is greater than that of a No. 25 or No. 30 (No. 3 or 4).

### Canal Irrigation

Irrigants are used to facilitate the cutting action of reamers and files and also to 'flush out' dentine debris and infected material. Some irrigants are used because they are able to dissolve and 'sterilize' inflamed or necrotic pulp tissue and dentine. Unfortunately the action of these irrigants is not selective, and if a solution can dissolve necrotic tissue it can effect the periodontal ligament and the peri-apical tissue as well if it is inadvertently pushed through the apical foramen. This results in a further inflammatory periapical reaction, which has to be resolved by the tissues. The use of such solutions would be acceptable if one could be certain that they would be confined within the root canal. Unfortunately this is not possible for even the gentlest and most delicate instrumentation within the canal results in a pumping action, which forces some (be it so minute) solution into the periapical tissue, with the inevitable after-pain or flare-up.

Further, some of the recommended irrigants are incompatible with the antibiotic pastes and these must be carefully removed before inserting dressings.

For these reasons it is suggested that the irrigant used be harmless to the periapical tissues, and sterile normal saline, water or local analgesic solution are considered the materials of choice.

It is convenient to irrigate canals by means of a hypodermic syringe and needle. However, unless great care is taken, it is possible to jam the needle tip against the canal wall, thus preventing flow back beside the needle and so forcing the solution through the apical foramen. A special endodontic syringe and needle* is available which minimizes this risk due to the stepped design of the needle tip. Unfortunately this needle is rather thick (gauge 23) and can only be used in canals of relatively large cross section.

Some operators prefer to use local analgesic solutions in cartridges because these are readily available, and can be used with fine gauge disposable needles which allows them to be passed closer to the apex with a lessened risk of jamming.

Hydrogen peroxide and sodium hypochlorite are two solutions favoured by many practitioners as root canal irrigants. They are used alternately and their interaction produces an effervescence of nascent oxygen and chlorine which forces debris out of the root canal. They are also said to soften and sterilize dentine. Their use as irrigants is questionable for hydrogen peroxide is a protoplasmic poison and Schilder and Amsterdam (1959) have shown that chlorinated soda is harmful to the eyes and subcutaneous connective tissues of the rabbit, and one can surmise that it will be injurious to the periapical tissues of humans as well. Blair (1970) and Bhat (1974) have described cases of emphysema attributable to the use of these drugs. Nicholls (1967) also warns that peroxide must be eliminated completely from the pulp cavity before it is sealed, since evolution of oxygen after sealing may force debris and micro-organisms into the periapical tissue.

### Canal Medication

It must be remembered that successful root canal therapy does not require the use of drugs and no amount of chemotherapy, unless accompanied by adequate mechanical débridement, will lead to a successful result. Several investigations have shown a successful outcome to root therapy where no medicaments were sealed in the root canal during treatment (Ingle and Zeldow, 1958; Grahnen and Krasse, 1963). Seltzer (1971) has pointed out that endodontists are preoccupied with the sterility of the root canal and with the drugs used to obtain sterility, and that this preoccupation has diverted attention from the more pertinent endodontic problem, i.e. the effect that these drugs have on the periapical tissues. Drugs potent enough to destroy bacteria may also destroy vital healthy periapical tissue, and in many instances the drug does more damage than the micro-organisms.

---

*Monojet Endodontic Syringe—502 ED: Sherwood Medical Industries Inc., 1831 Olive St., St. Louis, Missouri 63103.

Thus the ideal medicament used during root therapy should have the following properties:

1. Non-irritant to the periapical and periodontal tissues.
2. Able to eliminate or, at least, reduce the bacterial flora of the canal.
3. Prevent or lessen pain.
4. Reduce periapical inflammation.
5. Stimulate periapical repair.
6. Effective rapidly and active for long periods.
7. Capable of diffusion and penetration of dentine.
8. Effective in the presence of pus and organic debris.
9. Inexpensive and with a long shelf life.
10. Non-staining to either the soft tissue or to the tooth.

A medicament fulfilling all the above criteria is not yet available. Two groups of medicaments are currently in use: (1) The chemical antiseptics; (2) The antibiotics.

## 1. *The Chemical Antiseptics*

This group includes silver nitrate, iodine, phenol, formalin, various dyes, metacresyl acetate (cresatin); but these will not be discussed because they are rarely used.

*Camphorated para-monochlorophenol* (*CMCP*) has been used as a root canal medication since the nineteenth century and still enjoys considerable popularity in spite of its known toxic properties. It is made by mixing crystals of paramonochlorophenol with camphor. Harrison and Madonia (1970, 1971) studied the toxic properties of various materials by means of conjunctival inflammatory tests and intradermal injections into the abdomen of rabbits. Amongst the materials investigated were 35 per cent camphorated parachlorophenol (the preparation normally available) and 1 and 2 per cent aqueous parachlorophenol. They found that the CMCP was severely toxic and also coagulated protein. The 1 per cent aqueous MCP produced only a mild inflammatory reaction and there was no evidence of tissue necrosis.

Comparison of the effectiveness of these two materials showed that there was no basis for considering a 35 per cent concentration of CMCP as the optimum concentration for the antimicrobial effectiveness of the drug. They also showed that a 1 per cent concentration of parachlorophenol provides a ninefold increase beyond the effective *in vivo* concentration against most resistant organisms tested.

The dentinal tubules of teeth undergoing endodontic treatment have been shown to harbour micro-organisms and thus any medicament used to disinfect the root canal must be able to penetrate the tubules. The penetrability of aqueous and camphorated parachloro-phenol was investigated by Avny and his co-workers, in 1973, by means of autoradiographic studies. They found that aqueous parachlorophenol penetrated into the dentine from the pulp chamber and root canal and travelled at least to the cemento-dentinal junction, whereas camphorated parachlorophenol did not.

The other pertinent question often asked is whether the vapour from the material could adversely affect the periapical area, and if the vapour alone was sufficient to affect the bacterial flora within the root canal. Cwikla (1972), in a simple but effective *in vitro* experiment, showed that small amounts of medicaments (Formo-cresol, beechwood creosote, CMCP and Cresatin) placed on cotton-wool pellets and sealed in the pulp chamber of extracted human central incisors inhibited the growth of *Staphylococcus aureus* inoculated on agar plates and positioned some 1·5 mm above the apex of the teeth. The surface of the plate was, on average, 14·5 mm from the impregnated cotton pellets.

From these experiments it would seem that if these materials are used they must be used sparingly and with great care so as to minimize unpleasant symptoms.

APPLICATION OF CMCP

CMCP should be carried to the pulp cavity on a small pledget of cottonwool which has been squeezed nearly dry. The practice of either soaking a paper point in the medicament and placing it in the canal or of placing a dry paper point or cottonwool pledget in the cavity and then flooding with medicament, carried to the cavity by means of college tweezers, is dangerous because either the paper point itself or the medicament may pass through the apical foramen and cause pain or an acute flare up.

2. *The Antibiotics*

In spite of certain disadvantages combinations of antibiotics are closer to the ideal root canal medicament than the chemical anti-septics. This is so because they are virtually non-irritant to the periapical tissues, usually active in the presence of tissue fluids, and can be placed in the root canal in a vehicle that diffuses readily. Clinically, acute symptoms resolve more quickly following their use.

Medication with these drugs is criticized by some because, it is claimed, dangerous allergic reactions can occur during treatment and, also, because patients may build up a sensitivity to the drug which may cause problems if it is used on a later occasion. In spite of these criticisms the advantages of these medications far outweigh their disadvantages, and provided that the medicaments are confined to the root canal, sensitization and allergy reactions are extremely rare sequelae.

*Antibiotic Preparations Available*

Three preparations are currently available in the United Kingdom and these are the Boots* and 'P.D.' Polyantibiotic Root Canal Creams,† and 'Fokalmin' Endodontic Paste.‡

The Boots and 'P.D.' Creams are identical and are dispensed in cartridges. They have the following formula:

| | |
|---|---|
| Crystalline penicillin G | 150 000 units |
| Streptomycin (as sulphate) | 0·15 g |
| Chloramphenicol | 0·15 g |
| Sodium caprylate | 0·15 g |

in a silicone base containing barium sulphate. Unfortunately the base is not water-soluble and thus it is difficult to remove from root canals prior to root filling.

'Fokalmin' is available in a syringe supplied with plastic disposable needles. Its formula is more complex, the essential constituents being neomycin sulphate, chloramphenicol and prednisolone, in a water-soluble base.

The incorporation of the anti-inflammatory agent prednisolone is claimed to be an advantage, but this implies that if the agent is to be effective the paste must be forced periapically. Indeed, the instructions state that if periapical infection is present the paste should be pushed beyond the apex with sterile cottonwool or a paper point and, where required, it should be preceded by an incision so that the paste may be forced into the periapical region. This practice is of doubtful value, for besides irritating the tissues mechanically it is known that steroids interrupt the body's natural defence mechanism. This is brought about by reducing the permeability of small blood vessels, thus diminishing fluid exudate and the number of phagocytic cells. Granulating tissue formation is also inhibited.

Two other antibiotic pastes have been used at the Eastman Dental Hospital, Institute of Dental Surgery, with considerable success.

The first was commercially available until recently and was sold as Parke Davis Endodontic Compound, with the following formula:

| | |
|---|---|
| Chloramphenicol | 25 g |
| Nystatin | 5 g |
| Polyethylene glycol 4000 | 6 g |
| Polyethylene glycol 1500 | 40 g |
| Propylene glycol | 140 g |

---

*Boots Pure Drug Co., Nottingham, U.K.
†Produits Dentaires S.A., Vevey, Switzerland.
‡Lege Artis, Dental Manufacturing Co., D-7 Stuttgart 1, P.O. Box 992, West Germany.

111

The second formulation does not contain penicillin or chloramphenicol and consists of:

| | |
|---|---|
| Neomycin sulphate | 10·0 g |
| Polymyxin B sulphate | 3·0 Mega units |
| Bacitracin | 2·11 g |
| Nystatin | 2·5 Mega units |
| Polyethylene glycol 1300 | 25·6 g |
| Polyethylene glycol 1500 | 11·0 g |

Both these pastes can be dispensed by a pharmacist.

APPLICATION: The pastes are mechanically deposited within the canal by means of spiral root fillers (lentulo fillers) or, more safely, by means of hand reamers or files. It is also possible to inject the material into the root canal by means of specially designed syringes and needles. Great care must be exercised in using lentulo spirals, for these instruments are fragile and jam rather easily. The correct spiral, with regard to width, must be chosen and, as an added precaution, the length must be checked and marked on the spiral, so that the instrument can be placed in the canal about 1 mm short of the reamed length. The dental engine is started at the same time as the withdrawal of the instrument begins.

The use of pressure syringes and needles is also potentially dangerous because the needle may jam against the canal walls, and the paste be inadvertently forced into the periapical tissue.

A safer method may be to use a hand-held reamer or file smaller in size than the final instrument used to prepare the canal. Paste may be introduced into the canal and the walls thus coated with the antibiotic paste.

### The Sealing of the Medication (*Fig.* 57)

Irrespective of the medicament used care is required in sealing the access cavity, and ideally a double seal should be used. The medicament is first covered with a layer of dry cottonwool, followed by a small piece of warm gutta percha which is closely adapted to the access cavity walls. On cooling this forms the floor to a Black's Class I cavity, which is filled with a quick setting temporary filling. If possible the walls of the access cavity should be 'funnelled', so that masticatory pressures on the temporary filling do not dislodge the filling apically which may push the medicament within the root canal into the periapical tissue.

The advantages of an efficient double seal are twofold. Firstly, it ensures that no marginal leakage occurs with re-contamination of the pulp cavity. Indeed, some workers correctly consider this aspect of the treatment so important that they routinely use amalgam as a temporary filling material, because this gives the strongest and most efficient seal possible. It also prevents the accidental loss of the temporary seal which is embarrassing to the dentist and often uncomfortable for the patient. If the seal is lost the prepared root canal must be re-medicated and re-sealed, thus protracting the treatment.

Secondly, the use of a double seal ensures that, at the next visit, it is possible to remove the temporary seal from the access cavity without the risk of dropping or forcing small fragments of the material into the pulp cavity. The accidental blocking of a root canal complicates treatment because the blockage has to be cleared and this is a time consuming and, sometimes, an impossible operation.

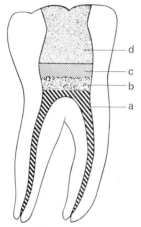

*Fig.* 57. The 'double' sealing of the medication. (*a*) Medicament, (*b*) cottonwool, (*c*) gutta percha, and (*d*) temporary filling which should be dense and placed in a 'funnelled' cavity so that it may better withstand the forces of mastication. There is no reason why amalgam cannot be used as a temporary seal.

The quick setting zinc oxide or amalgam layer is first removed so that the gutta percha is exposed. The access cavity is then cleared thoroughly until it is certain that there are no loose fragments within the cavity. The pulp cavity is next exposed by engaging the gutta percha and cottonwool with a No. 11 Briault probe and removing this secondary seal as one unit.

A further advantage of the double seal is that certain medicaments are incompatible with eugenol and if a quick setting zinc oxide is used it is separated from the medicament by the gutta percha.

There is no rule about how long a medicament should remain sealed before it is replaced. The drug's effectiveness will depend on how quickly it is diluted by the periapical exudate and/or inactivated by its interaction with the bacteria within the canal. Thus a tooth which is likely to produce considerable exudate should be re-dressed within 3 days. This is necessary not only to replace the inactive medicament but, more importantly, to remove the exudate which now fills the canal. If this is not done, pressure within the root canal will increase and the inflammatory symptoms and pain will return. If the periapical area of infection is inactive, the dressing may be left longer. Generally, medicaments become inactive after 2–3 weeks, probably the longest time that a dressing may be left sealed.

REFERENCES

Avny W. Y., Heiman G. R., Madonia J. V. and Wood N. K. (1973) Autoradiographic studies of the intracanal diffusion of aqueous and camphorated parachlorophenol in endodontics. *Oral Surg.* **36**, 80.

Bhat K. S. (1974) Tissue emphysema caused by hydrogen peroxide. *Oral Surg.* **38**, 304.

Blair G. S. (1970) Facial emphysema: An unusual dental hazard. *Dent. Mag. Oral Top.* **87**, 158.

Cwikla J. R. (1972) The vaporisation and capillarity effect of endodontic medicaments. *Oral Surg.* **34**, 117.

Grahnen H. and Krasse B. (1963) The effect of instrumentation and flushing of non-vital teeth in endodontic therapy. *Odontol. Revy* **14**, 167.

Harrison J. W. and Madonia J. V. (1970) Antimicrobial effectiveness of parachlorophenol. *Oral Surg.* **30**, 267.

Harrison J. W. and Madonia J. V. (1971) The toxicity of parachlorophenol. *Oral Surg.* **32**, 90.

Harty F. J., Parkins B. J. and Wengraf A. M. (1970) Success rate in root canal therapy: A retrospective study of conventional cases. *Br. Dent. J.* **128**, 65.

Harty F. J. and Stock C. J. R. (1974) The giromatic system compared with hand instrumentation in endodontics. *Br. Dent. J.* **137**, 239.

Ingle J. E. (1965) *Endodontics.* London, Kimpton, p. 201.

Ingle J. I. and Zeldow B. J. (1958) An evaluation of mechanical instrumentation and the negative culture in endodontic therapy. *J. Am. Dent. Assoc.* **57**, 471.

Jungmann C. L., Uchin R. A. and Bucher J. F. (1975) Effect of instrumentation on the shape of the root canal. *J. Endodont.* **1**, 66.

Nicholls E. (1967) *Endodontics.* Bristol, Wright, p. 125.

Renson C. E. (1971) An experimental study of the physical properties of human dentine. Ph.D. Thesis, University of London.

Seltzer S. (1971) *Endodontology: Biologic Considerations in Endodontic Procedures.* New York, McGraw-Hill.

Seltzer S., Bender I. B. and Turkenkopf S. (1963) Factors affecting successful repair after root canal therapy. *J. Am. Dent. Assoc.* **67**, 651.

Schilder H. and Amsterdam M. (1959) Inflammatory potential of root canal medicaments. *Oral Surg.* **12**, 211.

Vessey R. A. (1968) *The Effect of Filing versus Reaming on the Shape of the Prepared Root Canal.* Washington Bureau of Medicine, Navy Department.

CHAPTER 7

# CONVENTIONAL ROOT CANAL THERAPY II
## The Root Filling

THE root filling is intended to occlude the canal as well as adjacent canaliculi and tubules in order to prevent toxins and any organisms from getting into, or out of the canal. It should be noted that in order to do this it is only necessary to seal the apical portion of the canal unless there are patent lateral canals.

## CRITERIA FOR PLACING ROOT FILLINGS

Two criteria must be satisfied before the final filling of the root canal and these are: (1) The tooth must be symptomless; (2) The root canal must be dry.

A symptomless tooth implies that the patient is experiencing no discomfort and is able to bite on the tooth normally. The soft tissues above the apex are of normal colour and there is no apparent swelling. If a sinus were present preoperatively this should have healed. The tooth should not be in supra-occlusion and its mobility normal for the patient's dentition.

If any of the above symptoms are still present it is better if the tooth were re-dressed and kept under observation until completely symptomless.

The second criterion is more difficult to adhere to because periapical exudate into the canal may persist particularly in teeth with large apical foramina. In such cases and provided the tooth is otherwise symptomless, the canal is dried as well as possible with paper points and the root filling placed in the normal manner.

Some suggest the sealing of medicaments, such as zinc iodide-iodine solutions or 30 per cent hydrogen peroxide, within the canal in order to stop or diminish the periapical exudate (Grossman, 1974). As these materials are often irritating to the periapical tissues their use cannot be advocated.

A third criterion is often quoted as a prerequisite to root canal filling, i.e. negative *bacteriological culture*. This is a subject that has had an enormous influence on the development of root canal therapy, but its clinical usefulness is open to speculation. To culture a paper point taken from a canal is an easy enough matter but external contamination or poor sampling throw grave doubts upon the validity or significance of the results. Furthermore, where medicaments and especially the antibiotics have been used the sampling technique becomes even more open to criticism (Bender and Seltzer, 1963). Several surveys have shown that the results of root canal therapy, in the presence or absence of a sterile culture, are much the same (Bender and Seltzer, 1963; Seltzer et al., 1963; Morse, 1971). Thus the culturing of root canal contents remains a useful tool for research and as a teaching device in cleanliness, but it is less useful in routine root canal therapy.

There are rare cases of resistant and persistent infection in spite of adequate débridement and of conventional medication. In these cases the culturing of the canal contents is often useful in determining the pathogens present and their sensitivity to specific antibiotics and/or other medicaments.

## MATERIALS USED IN
## OBTURATING ROOT CANALS

It is probably true that no other hollow cavity in the body has been filled with as many materials as the root canal of a tooth (Rowe, 1968).

Ideally root filling materials should be:

1. Easily introduced into the root canal.

2. Not harmful to the periapical tissues or to the tooth.

3. Plastic on insertion but able to set to a solid shortly after, preferably with a degree of expansion.

4. Stable, i.e. they must not resorb, shrink, or be affected by moisture.

5. Adherent to the canal walls.

6. Self-sterilizing and bacteriostatic.

7. Radio-opaque.

8. Inexpensive and with a long shelf life.

9. Easily removed if necessary.

The ideal material has not been discovered and it is usually necessary to use a combination of materials and these are given in *Table* 1.

*Table* 1

| | | |
|---|---|---|
| 1. Cements | Alone or with obturating points | a. Silver |
| 2. Plastics | | b. Gutta Percha |
| 3. Resorbable pastes | | c. Plastic |
| 4. Gutta Percha with Solvents | | |
| 5. Amalgam | | |

## 1. Cements

Cements include zinc phosphate, plaster-of-Paris, ethoxybenzoic acid (EBA) cement, and more commonly, modifications of zinc oxide-eugenol.

Most of the recommended zinc-oxide/eugenol cements are based on the following formula given by Rickert and Dixon (1931) and Dixon and Rickert (1938)

*Powder*
| | |
|---|---|
| Zinc oxide | 41·2 g |
| Precipitated silver | 30·0 g |
| White rosin | 16·0 g |
| Thymol iodide | 12·8 g |

*Liquid*
| | |
|---|---|
| Oil of cloves | 78·0 ml |
| Canada balsam | 22·0 ml |

This cement has been used satisfactorily for many years because of its good handling and sealing properties. It suffers from a serious disadvantage in that the precipitated silver, added for its bacteriostatic properties, stains the dentinal tubules.

To overcome this problem Grossman, in 1958, modified the formula thus:

*Powder*
| | |
|---|---|
| Zinc oxide | 42 parts |
| Staybelite resin | 27 parts |
| Bismuth subcarbonate | 15 parts |
| Barium sulphate | 15 parts |
| Sodium borate anhydrous | 1 part |

*Liquid*
Eugenol

Both of these cements are available commercially or can be dispensed by a pharmacist. Both have a slight disadvantage in that the resin is of coarse particle size and unless the material is spatulated vigorously during mixing an uncrushed piece of resin may lodge on the wall of the canal and prevent the root filling point from seating at the correct level during insertion. A preferable cement may be 'Tubli-Seal'* marketed as a two paste system and thus easy to mix into a smooth grit-free paste.

Two other cements must be mentioned as they are in common use. These are 'N2 Normal'† and 'Endomethasone'.‡ Both contain a proportion of paraformaldehyde which if accidentally deposited in the periapical tissue may give rise to a severe inflammatory reaction (Keresztesi and Kellner, 1966; Friend and Browne, 1968; Grieve and Parkholm, 1973).

---

*'Tubli-Seal', Kerr Manufacturing Company, Detroit 8, Michigan, U.S.A.
†'N2 Normal', AGSA, Switzerland.
‡'Endomethasone', Specialités Septodont, 29 Rue des Petites-Écuries, Paris (10e),

Endomethasone has the following formula:

| | |
|---|---|
| Dexamethasone | 0·01 g |
| Hydrocortisone acetate | 1·0  g |
| Di-Iodothymol | 25·0  g |
| Trioxymethylene (i.e. paraformaldehyde) | 2·20 g |
| Expedient q.s. | 100·0 g |

Sometimes an Endomethasone root filling gives rise to pain or discomfort some 6–8 weeks after insertion. One can postulate that this occurs because the corticosteroid masks any inflammatory reaction until it is, itself, removed from the area. Presumably the trioxymethylene (which is a synonym for 'paraformaldehyde') is not resorbed equally quickly and the symptoms of the inflammatory reaction become apparent.

## 2. Plastics

In this modern age of plastics it was inevitable that these materials would, sooner or later, be utilized as root fillings. Two such materials are AH26* and 'Diaket'†. The former was introduced by Schroeder (1957) and consisted of an epoxy resin base with a bisphenol diglycidyl ether liquid.

Diaket is marketed as Normal or Diaket-A. Both are essentially a polyvinyl resin in a polyketone vehicle and the latter has a proportion of hexachlorophene to enhance its disinfecting properties. It is claimed that these materials harden with negligible contraction and have a degree of adhesion towards dentine.

Experimental tissue reaction studies are confusing, but it is generally agreed that there is an initial severe inflammatory reaction which subsides after some weeks. Controlled human studies are few but the consensus of opinion is that these materials are reasonably well tolerated by the periapical tissues. Clinically, the setting time of root filling materials is important because the root filling point may have to be adjusted following radiographic check. AH26 sets extremely slowly—in about 48 hours. Diaket, on the other hand, sets in about 5 minutes on the slab and even more rapidly in the mouth.

## 3. Resorbable Pastes

Virtually all root filling materials, including metals, are to a greater or lesser degree resorbed if implanted in the periapical tissue. By common usage the term *Resorbable paste* refers to those pastes which never set on being introduced into the root canal and are speedily removed from the periapical tissue by phagocytosis.

---

*Amalgamated Dental, 26–40 Broadwick Street, London, W1.
†ESPE Gmbh, Seefeld, Oberbayern, West Germany.

*Iodoform* was used, in general surgery, as an antiseptic which promoted granulation tissue long before it was introduced as a root filling material by Walkhoff in 1882. The medicament still enjoys considerable popularity and is available commercially as 'Kri-I' paste* which consists of—

| | |
|---|---|
| Parachlorophenol | 45 parts |
| Camphor | 49 parts |
| Menthol | 6 parts |

This is mixed with iodoform powder in a ratio of 40 : 60 to give a thick yellow paste with a characteristic odour.

Kri-I paste is used both as an antiseptic dressing and as the final root filling. In teeth with a necrotic pulp it is suggested that the material be forced into the periapical tissues in order to 'sterilize' them. If a sinus is present the paste is injected into the canal and forced past the apical foramen until it oozes out of the sinus.

The paste has been investigated by many including Castagnola and Orlay (1952), Laws (1964) and Bell (1969). They agree that it is rapidly removed from the tissues by macrophage action and that there occurs an initial severe inflammatory reaction which subsides after about 3 months. Radiographically the paste disappears, in a much shorter period, not only from the periapical tissues but also from the apical portion of the root canal. It is said that the paste is replaced by granulation tissue and that there is an ingrowth of periodontal tissue into the root canal.

The technique can be criticized in that the forcing of paste into the periapical tissues may introduce infected material from the root canal into an area that is normally sterile. Further, the paste, being rapidly resorbable, does not afford an effective apical seal.

Bell (1969) has succinctly summarized the position, by stating that, 'there is no doubt that when used for root fillings Kri-I paste does produce acceptable results in a percentage of cases (68·2 per cent). However, from the results of the experiments, it would appear likely that clinical success occurs in spite of, rather than because of, the Kri-I paste'.

### 4. *Obturating Points*

It is generally recognized that cements and pastes cannot be used alone because they form an inadequate seal against the irregular canal walls. To obtain an adequate seal it is necessary to force the cement against the root canal walls and this is usually achieved by using gutta percha or silver points.

Plastic points are also available but these are not popular because they are brittle, and have no advantage over conventional points.

---

*'Kri-I' Paste—Pharmachemie AG Zurich 53, Switzerland.

Studies have also been carried out to check the sealing properties of gutta percha or silver points used without sealer (Marshall and Massler, 1961; Kapsimalis and Evans, 1966; Talim and Singh, 1967). All agree that the use of a sealer is essential for effective canal obturation.

Agreement, however, ceases here and some endodontists are currently debating the relative merits of one material over the other. Some feel that their chosen material is the only one which results in satisfactory root fillings and condemn the use of all other materials. This attitude is to be deprecated for gutta percha and silver points have different properties, which makes each eminently suitable in different situations.

SILVER POINTS: These are rigid in small diameters and can readily negotiate curves in fine canals. Because of their rigidity and radio-opacity they can be placed accurately in the root canal. Provided they are covered by sealer they are stable. Luks (1965) and Harris (1971) have reported cases of rusting of silver points within the canal but this will only happen if the point is loose within the canal and inadequately covered by sealer and thus not attached to the canal wall by the cement. If the point impinges on the periapical tissue any sealer that may be covering the point is rapidly resorbed and the point rusts.

GUTTA PERCHA POINTS: These are difficult to use, particularly in the smaller diameters, because they are not rigid and they buckle easily. Gutta percha is generally considered inert, but Feldmann and Nyborg (1962) and Seltzer et al. (1969) question this.

The main claimed advantage of gutta percha points lies in their compressibility, which enables them to be adapted closely to the irregular wall of the root canal. Another claimed advantage is that the material is soluble in chloroform, ether, xylol and, less so, in eugenol, and thus can be removed from the canal should this become necessary.

GUTTA PERCHA WITH SOLVENTS: It is suggested that better condensation and adhesion to the canal walls can be obtained if gutta percha is used in conjunction with one of the solvents mentioned above. This technique gives excellent results in expert hands, but has been criticized because the solvents used are volatile and the root filling shrinks as the solvent evaporates. There is a danger that if the canal is overfilled the chloroform in the mixture may cause periapical tissue damage because it is a fairly powerful irritant and is also cytotoxic (Kawahara et al., 1968).

## 5. *Amalgam*

This material has been used extensively as the root filling of choice prior to apicectomy and also as a seal in the retrograde root filling technique (*see* Chapter 8) (Messing, 1958; Herd, 1968; Harty et al., 1970a; Hill, 1970).

The use of amalgam for conventional root filling has not been reported and this is strange for of all the materials readily available to the dental surgeon this is the one he uses most frequently with best results in everyday practice. If one considers the ideal properties of root filling materials (p. 116) it is seen that it fulfils most of the prerequisites.

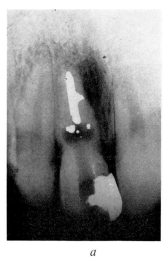 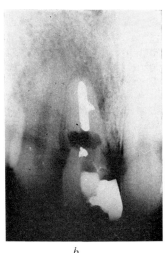

*a*           *b*

*Fig.* 58. *a*, Amalgam root filling showing the ease with which it can be condensed into irregular areas. *b*, Radiograph showing resolution of lateral radiolucent area 12 months after insertion of amalgam root filling. (*Courtesy of Mr. T. R. Hill.*)

The set material is stable and probably the only available root filling that is truly non-resorbable. It is radio-opaque, inexpensive and has a long shelf life. It is plastic on insertion and sets reasonably quickly. The plasticity of the material allows it to be condensed into irregular areas of root canal and also into accessory and lateral canals of moderate diameter (*Fig.* 58). Because of the presence of moisture within the root canal amalgam expands slightly on setting and this must enhance the efficacy of the apical seal.

Until recently it could only be used in relatively straight canals of large diameter. However, it is now possible to use the material in canals that can be reamed to a No. 40 reamer (*see* Technique, p. 127).

The only disadvantage is that it can not be removed easily from the canal should this become necessary. However, lack of apical seal is, without a doubt, the chief cause of root canal therapy failure. Amalgam root filling gives the best possible seal and the number of failures is very small. If an amalgam root filling fails it is possible to salvage the tooth by means of apicectomy, where it is the root filling of choice because it can not be disturbed during resection.

Friend and Browne (1968) have shown that the material is well tolerated by the periapical tissues when fully set, and this is confirmed by the large number of patients seen where amalgam has been inadvertently left in the tissues after apicectomy. In these cases healing has taken place around the amalgam particles without any postoperative symptoms except for the occasional tattooing of the mucosa. When amalgam is used for conventional root therapy no periapical irritation occurs because the amalgam is confined within the root canal and does not come into contact with the periapical tissues.

Amalgam has been used for some years by colleagues and the author at the Institute of Dental Surgery, and a long term clinical evaluation is continuing.

## ROOT FILLING TECHNIQUES

There are two commonly used techniques, i.e.: (*a*) The sectional or split cone root filling; (*b*) The complete obturation of the canal.

Irrespective of the technique used the main purpose of the operation must be kept in mind, i.e. that the root canal should be hermetically sealed from the peridental tissues. Lack of adequate seal is the principal cause of endodontic failure.

### I. *The Apical 1/5th, sectional, or 'split cone' technique*

In this technique only the apical 3 or 4 mm is filled and it is particularly useful in teeth with straight root canals which could conceivably ever be used for a post-retained restoration. The practice of filling such canals completely and subsequently removing part of the root filling to accommodate a post is fraught with danger because of the possibility of root perforation and the risk of disturbing the all important apical seal. Neagley (1969) showed that if canals were instrumented subsequent to root filling the seal was disturbed in a high percentage of cases. In his experiments the full silver point root filling was found to be the most vulnerable with 88 per cent seal breakdown. However, when a sectional technique was used and the root filling was *not* disturbed by the cutting instrument, the canal was as well sealed as in the control specimens. Laterally condensed and warm gutta percha techniques gave better results with only

21 per cent of apical seal disturbance. Presumably if these materials had been used as sectional root fillings and *not* disturbed by the cutting instrument the seal would not have been affected.

The materials commonly used in this technique are silver or gutta percha points in combination with sealer. Recently amalgam alone has also been advocated.

### 1. *Sectional Silver Point Technique*

It is important that the correct size of point is selected and the tip of the point fits the apical portion of the canal snugly. Ideally it should be possible to select a standardized silver point which fits accurately a canal prepared with a matched standardized reamer. The specifications suggested by the International Standards Organization state that a silver point of a certain number should have a diameter 9 microns less than the equivalent numbered reamer. Unfortunately this very stringent requirement has not been achieved by manufacturers and it is still necessary to select the point by trial and error (Harty and Sondoozi, 1972).

The selected point must be a tight fit in the apical 3 or 4 mm but must fit loosely in the coronal portion of the root canal, so that the fit of the apical section can be evaluated. Thus it may be necessary to thin the coronal portion of the point with sandpaper discs. This is easily done by mounting, face to face, on a mandrel, two 7/8 inch sandpaper discs. With the engine revolving slowly, the point to be reshaped (held in haemostats) is inserted and rotated between the faces of the discs.

If the point is to fit properly a slight positive pressure will be required to seat it home fully, and there must be some resistance to its withdrawal. At this stage a diagnostic radiograph should be taken to check the position of the point relative to the radiographic apex.

The point should be removed from the root canal with locked haemostats placed level with a fixed point on the tooth, e.g. the incisal edge.

If the radiograph shows an unsatisfactory point placement the apical section must either be thinned or a smaller point selected and the whole procedure repeated and checked. Sometimes, particularly with the larger sizes of silver point, the tip shape of the point does not match the prepared apical area of the root canal because of manufacturing discrepancies. In such cases the tip of the silver point should be shaped to match the tip of the reamer used to prepare the canal (*Fig.* 59).

The point is again removed from the canal with locked artery forceps. It is then notched with a carborundum disc at a point 3–4 mm from the tip until only a thin segment of metal connects the apical portion to the main part of the point. Alternatively the point may be grooved all the way around its circumference until a fine isthmus only connects the two parts of the point (*Fig.* 60).

The point, still firmly held in the haemostats, is disinfected in 70 per cent isopropyl alcohol, dried and placed to one side.

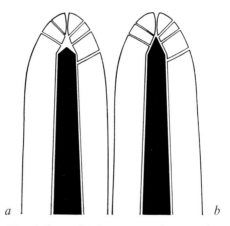

*Fig.* 59. *a*, Tip of silver point does not match prepared root canal. *b*, Re-shaped silver point seated at correct level.

The canal is carefully dried with paper points and the apical portion lightly coated with the root sealer of choice which is carried into position with a lentulo spiral filler or with a reamer or file. If a filler is used great care must be exercised so that the filler does not accidentally jam and fracture within the canal (*see* p. 74). It must also be remembered that because of the considerable forward propelling force created by the rotating spiral filler sealer may be forced through an apical foramen not already 'sealed' with dentine grindings. Care must also be taken not to deposit too much paste in the apical portion of the root canal for this excess paste will either prevent the obturating point from seating at the correct level or be forced through the apical foramen by the piston effect of the point on the sealer. If too much paste has been deposited within the root canal the excess must be removed either with a reamer or with a counter clockwise rotating spiral filler, placed 2 mm short of the reamed length, again with the same precautions as when introducing the sealer.

Because of the danger of spiral filler fracture it may be safer if sealer paste is introduced into the root canal with a hand held reamer of slightly smaller diameter than the final instrument used in preparing the root canal.

When the sealer is in position the prepared silver point is lightly coated with sealer and gently introduced into the canal until the correct level is reached as evidenced by the position of the locked artery forceps.

The apical portion now has to be severed from the main part of the silver point and this is achieved by moving the artery forceps

*Fig.* 60. Methods of sectioning silver points for use in sectional root filling techniques.

0·5–1 mm away from the tooth surface, regripping the silver point and, whilst applying an apical pressure on the point, rotating the forceps about the point until the apical portion is severed and left in situ.

A final diagnostic radiograph may now be taken, the empty portion of the canal walls cleaned of sealer with chloroform or xylol and the coronal access cavity sealed either temporarily or permanently.

### 2. *Messing Precision Apical Silver Point Technique*

The foregoing technique suffers from one disadvantage due to the malleability of silver which sometimes prevents the breaking of the silver point in situ despite careful grooving at the site of the projected breakage point.

To overcome this problem Messing (1969) suggested the manufacture of apical silver cones carrying a screw thread to engage in hollow cylindrical shafts attached to a handle. He also suggested that the cones should be standardized and matched to standard reamers and files.

125

These cones are now available as 'P.D.' Apical Silver Tips* in 3 and 5 mm lengths and 12 I.S.O. standardized sizes (Nos. 45–140). Matching handles are also available and these now have the added advantage in being adjustable with regard to overall length, thus obviating the necessity of marking the length of the prepared canal onto the shaft of the instrument (*Fig.* 61).

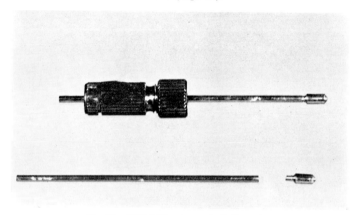

*Fig.* 61. 'P.D.' Messing apical silver tips.

The *method of use* is simple and has some advantages over the conventional sectional silver point technique. A sterile point is selected which matches the last reamer used in enlarging the canal. This is screwed onto the shaft and the handle is adjusted to the length of the prepared canal. The assembled point and handle are then introduced into the canal until the handle stop is coincident with the incisal edge or cusp-tip. It is important that the tip is not forced into the canal and it may be necessary to enlarge the canal by further reaming. The point is deemed to fit correctly when it reaches to within 1 mm from the radiographic apex of the tooth and demonstrates a 'tug-back' resistance on being removed from the canal. The canal is then dried and sealer introduced as before. The handle is then unscrewed whilst exerting a gentle but firm apical pressure. As the thread finally disengages, a click will be heard and a slight jar will be apparent to the fingers holding the handle which may then be withdrawn leaving the apical sectional filling in situ.

This technique has a further advantage in that the cone can often be removed from the canal should this be necessary subsequently. This is done by selecting the appropriate handle, inserting it in the canal and re-engaging the threads of the cone and withdrawing the point.

*Produits Dentaires S.A., Vevey, Switzerland.

The tips and handles can be sterilized by dry heat, autoclaving or chemically, but Messing (1975) warns that if chemical sterilization is used the cones and handles should not be joined and left immersed in sterilizing solution for long periods as electrolytic action may damage the fine threads. He suggests that they be sterilized, dried and stored separately.

### 3. Sectional Gutta Percha Point Technique

This technique is similar to the sectional silver point technique in its preliminary stages, i.e. in selection, trial fit and radiographic check. The technique differs in the method of sectioning and carriage into the root canal.

The selected gutta percha point is sectioned, with a scalpel blade, some 3–4 mm from its tip. This small piece is attached to a straight root canal plugger or to a length of stainless-steel wire, of lesser diameter than the gutta percha point, by gently heating the wire and pressing the end against the cut portion. A mark is then placed on the wire so that the gutta percha plus wire length equals the length of the prepared canal.

The canal walls and the gutta percha point are coated with sealer as before and the stainless-steel wire with attached point is introduced into the root canal until the correct level is reached. The sectional point is disengaged from the wire by gently pushing apically and, at the same time, twisting the wire.

### 4. Sectional Amalgam Root Filling Technique

The advantages of amalgam as a root filling material have been discussed on p. 121.

Whilst it is technically possible to place amalgam in the apical area of the root canal with root canal pluggers, the operation is greatly facilitated by the use of one of the three commercially available endodontic amalgam carriers. These are essentially similar in design but vary in size. Their construction has been described on p. 86. The Messing and Hill carriers are of relatively wide diameter and were primarily designed for the root filling of anterior teeth prior to or during apicectomy.

The Dimashkieh carrier (*Fig.* 43, p. 86) is smaller and more delicate and is particularly useful in the root filling of teeth with fine canals and in posterior teeth whose root canals can be reamed to No. 40. Because of its fine diameter the shaft of the instrument is flexible and can be used in canals of moderate curvature.

The amalgam is mixed in a 1 : 1 proportion and is not squeezed dry. Prior to use the shaft of the carrier is marked with marking paste or with a rubber stop at a point equal to the length of the prepared root canal. Small increments of amalgam are picked up with the carrier and introduced into the root canal until the mark on the shaft coincides with the reference point on the tooth. Care must be taken not to depress the plunger, which discharges the amalgam, until the tip of the instrument is at the correct level. If doubt exists about the position of the instrument relative to the apex a diagnostic X-ray can be taken to ensure that the carrier is at the correct level.

The amalgam is deposited by depressing the plunger and condensed with a fine root canal plugger or with a length of stainless-steel wire of suitable diameter. Further increments of amalgam are deposited and condensed so that the completed root filling obturates 2–3 mm of the root canal. It should be noted that sealer is not used in this technique and the amalgam alone forms the root filling.

A criticism of this technique may be that the vertical pressure exerted during condensation of the amalgam might force the material, or free mercury, through the apical foramen. Provided the canal has been prepared satisfactorily, that is, the apical foramen has not been breached and instrumentation confined to within 1 mm of the apical foramen, it is unlikely that the amalgam can be forced past the apical constriction.

The only occasion when mercury rich amalgam can be pushed into the periodontal tissues occurs when there exists an accessory or lateral canal, of relatively wide diameter, at some distance from the apical foramen. This is so because condensation of several amalgam increments results in a softer, mercury rich layer on the coronal aspect of the root filling. This soft layer of amalgam can be forced laterally so as to partly occlude the accessory canal. However, clinically it is not possible to use vertical pressures of sufficient magnitude to force the soft amalgam or mercury laterally into the periodontal tissues.

As has already been mentioned the chief disadvantage of this technique is that the root filling cannot be easily removed if the treatment fails. This criticism can be made for nearly all sectional techniques, but if one believes in the importance of the seal at the apex then the risk of failure would seem to be lessened because of the improved seal obtained with amalgam.

## II. *Complete Obturation of the Root Canal*

Ideally the entire pulp cavity should be mechanically cleaned, sterilized and obliterated so that no space exists for the accumulation of tissue fluids, bacteria or their degradation products.

If one were certain that the pulp cavity was always a tube with an opening at either end then the sectional technique could be employed in all cases. However, anatomical studies show that whilst accessory canals are relatively rare in single rooted teeth, lateral canals frequently occur in multi-rooted teeth (Hess and Zurcher, 1925; Kramer, 1960; Lowman et al., 1973).

For this reason and also because post crowns are not usually constructed in posterior teeth the pulp cavities of multi-rooted teeth should be filled completely.

The techniques used in such cases are:

1. Silver points and sealer
2. Techniques with gutta percha
   a. Single cone gutta percha
   b. Laterally condensed gutta percha
   c. Vertically condensed warm gutta percha
   d. Gutta percha with solvents
3. Sealer 'pastes' used alone.

### 1. *Silver Points and Sealer*

Silver points were originally introduced by Jasper in 1933 and since then have had a chequered career as root filling materials. Nevertheless, their comparative rigidity and ease in negotiating fine curved canals makes them ideal for use in posterior teeth where the use of gutta percha or amalgam is almost impossible even in expert hands.

However, it is important to realize that the point is not the root filling but rather than it acts as 'spreader' for the sealer which is the actual root filling providing the hermetic seal to the root canal. The use of silver points without cement is doomed to failure as has been demonstrated by Marshall and Massler (1961), Kapsimalis and Evans (1966) and Talim and Singh (1967).

The selection and fit of the silver point is identical to the sectional technique discussed on p. 123. The point should pass loosely through the coronal and middle third of the root canal and should bind snugly in the apical third only. When this is achieved a check X-ray is taken and the point removed from the canal with locked artery forceps so that it may be subsequently replaced in the canal to exactly the same level.

The point is then grooved with a separating disc at a level which will allow fracture 3–4 mm coronally to the floor of the pulp chamber. This level is chosen so that a portion of the silver point is readily visible and available for adjustment or even for removal should it become necessary (*Fig.* 62). If other canals are present they are filled in turn with silver points if of fine diameter, or with gutta percha if of a large size.

Because lateral canals occur most frequently in the furcation areas of multi-rooted teeth it is essential that the space around the loosely fitting silver point in the middle and coronal thirds of the root canal and the pulp chamber floor be obliterated as well as the apical third and foramen. This is achieved by laterally condensing fine gutta percha points around the master silver point in the manner described under the lateral condensation technique below. When this is complete the floor of the pulp chamber is coated with sealer and the 'tails' of the gutta percha points extruding from the root canals folded and condensed firmly against the floor with a warmed amalgam plugger. This should result in a thin layer of gutta percha lying flat against the floor of the pulp chamber with the coronal portions of the silver points passing through the condensed gutta percha.

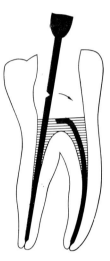

*Fig.* 62. Partially completed root filling using silver points. Note that gutta percha has been condensed around the points, in the coronal third of the root and on the floor of the pulp chamber. The point in the mesial canal has been notched and fractured and the end folded into the mass of the gutta percha.

Root filling the floor of the pulp chamber of multi-rooted teeth is very important for, as has already been seen, lateral canals are present in a percentage of specimens (*Fig.* 63). Failure to seal these canals may lead to inadequate treatment from an endodontic viewpoint or because of periodontal complications (*see* Chapter 10).

The silver points are now fractured at the grooved level by bending the free end backwards and forwards. This end is then folded so that it lies flat against the gutta percha base and this is achieved with the aid of a serrated amalgam plugger or, in difficult cases, by using the bending tool supplied for use with T.M.S. screws.*

When the free ends of all points are bent so that they lie flat against the gutta percha base a further thin layer of pink gutta percha is condensed above the points (*Fig.* 63). This precaution is taken so that should it become necessary to re-instrument the canal

*Whaledent Inc., 304 Ashland Place, Brooklyn, New York 11217.

due to failure of the root filling it is a relatively simple procedure to remove the access cavity filling to the level of the pink gutta percha, without cutting or disturbing the silver points. Once the level of the gutta percha root filling has been demonstrated it is relatively easy to remove the gutta percha with hand instruments, straighten the silver points and remove them from the canal with fine beaked haemostats or with Steiglitz forceps (*see* Chapter 5).

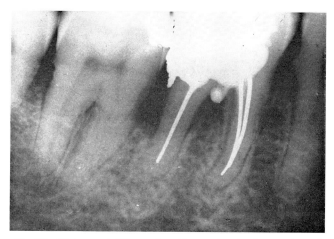

*Fig.* 63. Molar root filling using silver points in the canals and condensed gutta percha in coronal third and floor of pulp chamber. The extruded sealer in furcation area is evidence of a lateral canal.

## 2. Techniques with Gutta Percha

*a.* SINGLE GUTTA PERCHA CONE METHOD: The advocates of this technique suggest that with the introductions of standardized root canal instruments and matching silver and gutta percha points it is possible to prepare a canal to a standard size and obturate it with a standard cone (Grossman, 1974).

The technique is simple and consists of matching a standard point to the prepared canal as observed on the X-ray and to the last reamer used in preparing the canal. The cone is marked at a point equal to the known instrumented length of the root canal. It is then tried in the canal and if the mark corresponds to the incisal or occlusal reference point it is assumed that the tip is at the correct level, and this is checked radiographically. If the point does not reach the apex, the canal is enlarged slightly or a new smaller point selected. If it is through the apical foramen a portion is cut off corresponding to the length past the apical foramen.

When it is certain that the point fits snugly at the correct level, the walls of the root canal are coated lightly with cement, the point

131

itself is 'buttered' in cement and passed into the root canal until the mark on the point coincides with the incisal or occlusal fixed point of reference.

This technique has several disadvantages and cannot be considered as one that obturates completely the pulp cavity. Root canals are seldom round throughout their length except possibly at the apical 2 or 3 mm. Thus it is almost always impossible to prepare a canal to a round cross section throughout its length. Further, it has been shown that matched endodontic instruments, silver points and, more particularly, gutta percha points have not yet been manufactured to acceptable limits (Harty and Sondoozi, 1972).

For these reasons the single gutta percha point technique, at best, only seals the root canal in the apical 2 or 3 mm and can be considered no better than the sectional technique. Further if a post retained restoration has to be constructed it is almost certain that the post preparation will disturb not only the coronal and middle third portions of the gutta percha point but also the apical section (Neagley, 1969). This accidental dislodgement of the apical section occurs because the bulk of the point is loose within the canal and the post preparing instrument (be it hand held or engine driven) entwines itself around the loose point and usually removes it entirely on withdrawal.

*b.* LATERALLY CONDENSED GUTTA PERCHA: This technique is an extension of the single cone technique and accepts the fact that a single cone only fits accurately in the apical 2 or 3 mm. An attempt is then made to obturate the unfilled spaces around the primary gutta percha master point with additional secondary points. These are condensed, without heat, against the master point. Protagonists of this technique assume that it is possible to compress gutta percha by pressure alone so that the spaces between individual points are obliterated.

Schilder et al. (1974) dispute this and state that gutta percha is less compressible than water. They suggest that the reduction in apparent volume which takes place as a result of mechanical manipulation is due to collapse of internal voids and occurs well within the compaction forces. Brayton et al. (1973) evaluated the lateral condensation technique by decalcifying 87 extracted teeth that had been filled with this method and found considerable variations between the radiographic appearance of the root filling and the actual state of the 'condensed' points which were irregular in form and condensation. They also found that there was inadequate sealer dispersal.

In spite of these criticisms the technique is useful in wide oval canals and particularly where it is suspected that lateral or accessory canals exist.

The initial stages of the technique are the same as the single cone technique, i.e. a master point is selected so that it fits accurately and tightly in the apical 2 or 3 mm. The apical level of the master cone should be 0·5–1 mm shorter than the final level to which the cone will ultimately be seated. This is necessary because the vertical pressure used in condensing the gutta percha tends to force the apical portion of the point in an apical direction and if the master point is very close to the apical foramen there is a danger of over-filling.

When the master point is in position specially designed 'spreaders', such as the Kerr,* 'Starlite'† or Luks‡ instruments are placed in the canal as far apically as possible and the master point is condensed laterally against the canal walls. The pressure is applied several times and the gutta percha kept under pressure for about 15 seconds.

The spreader is then rapidly withdrawn and replaced with a gutta percha point, lightly coated with sealer, of the same shape and general dimensions as the spreader. The procedure is repeated until no more points can be wedged into the canal. The coronal excess is removed with a hot instrument and the access cavity filled with a suitable permanent or temporary filling.

The advantage of this technique is that the canal is filled with a seemingly dense, dimensionally stable root filling, which is less likely to be disturbed than a single cone filling if a post retained restoration is required at a later date.

However, as Schilder (1967) has pointed out, the root filling does not consist of a homogeneous mass of material, but rather of a large number of individual gutta percha points tightly pressed together and joined by a frictional grip and cementing substance. The only area where true homogeneity exists is in the coronal section where the coronal excess has been fused together with the hot instrument.

By the very nature of the technique the greatest density of gutta percha exists in the coronal portion of the canal and the filling is progressively less dense apically. Indeed, the all important apical 2–3 mm is obturated with a single cone only, as in the sectional and single cone techniques.

It is true that the initial postoperative radiograph often shows lateral canals apparently well filled with filling material but this can only be sealer for it is not possible to condense gutta percha into such fine canals. Often this sealer is resorbed quickly as shown in subsequent postoperative radiographs (*Fig.* 64).

In spite of the above criticisms the technique has been used for many years with considerable success.

---

*Kerr Manufacturing Co., Detroit 8, Michigan, U.S.A.
†Star Dental Mfg Co. Inc., Philadelphia, Pa. 19139, U.S.A.
‡Luks Root Canal Pluggers, Union Broach Co. Inc., 45–18 Court Square, Long Island City, New York 11101, U.S.A.

*c.* VERTICALLY CONDENSED WARM GUTTA PERCHA: This technique has been developed by Schilder (1967) in an attempt to overcome the deficiencies of the lateral condensation technique. It aims at using heat to render gutta percha plastic which is then condensed vertically thus creating a homogeneous root filling of greater density throughout the canal but particularly in the apical area. The instrumentation required differs from that of the preceding technique and consists of one pointed root canal spreader which Schilder has renamed a 'heat carrier'. This instrument is the only one that is actually heated. Condensation is effected with a graded series of pluggers which are tapering but differ from conventional spreaders in being blunt-ended. The pluggers have been further refined by having score lines at 5-mm intervals. They are available in 8 sizes.*

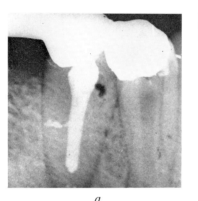 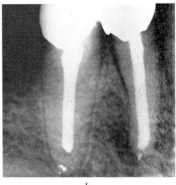

*a*           *b*

*Fig.* 64. *a*, Postoperative radiograph showing apparently well filled lateral canal. *b*, Radiograph 14 days later showing resorption of sealer from lateral canal.

A master cone is fitted and checked as in the preceding techniques paying particular attention to the selection of a cone that is wider apically than is the root canal. A small amount of sealer is introduced into the apical portion of the canal with a hand held spiral root filler and the master cone placed in position. The coronal end of the cone is then severed with a hot instrument and the warm end remaining within the canal folded and packed into the pulp chamber with a large plugger. The heat carrier is then heated to cherry redness and plunged into the gutta percha to a depth of 3–4 mm. As soon as the gutta percha is plastic the heat carrier is removed and the softened material is condensed, in an apical direction, with a suitable plugger.

*Star Dental Mfg Co. Inc., Philadelphia, Pa. 19139, U.S.A.

The use of a spreader heated to cherry redness is sometimes viewed apprehensively by both patient and operator but Marlin and Schilder (1973) have shown that because of the low thermal conductivity of gutta percha the temperature increase within the root canal was 4° C in the apical region and 12·5° C in the body of the preparation and thus did not constitute a danger to the patient.

The heating and condensing procedure is repeated until the coronal third of the canal is filled laterally and vertically. At this stage neither the apical nor middle-thirds of the root canal have been affected and in order to reach these areas gutta percha now has to be removed from the centre of the gutta percha filling. This is carried out with the heated spreader which is forced deeper into the canal. Gutta percha is removed from the canal as it adheres to the instrument. The remaining gutta percha is gradually condensed vertically and laterally until the walls of the canal are coated with a thin layer of material.

In this manner the apical area is reached where the gutta percha is heated and condensed in the same way. The score lines on the pluggers give a useful indication of the depth of condensation.

At this stage the root canal is essentially empty except for the apical 2 or 3 mm and the thin coating of gutta percha on the walls. The remaining portion of the canal is filled with small increments of gutta percha (about 2–3 mm²) which are heated and condensed vertically as before. No cement is used at this stage and the canal is filled completely and three dimensionally by gutta percha alone.

Schilder agrees that even with this refined root filling technique it is unlikely that lateral canals are filled with gutta percha but rather with cement alone which is extruded into the fine canals by the pressure of the condensed gutta percha.

The technique has much to commend it and there is no doubt that the resultant root filling is homogeneous, dense and fills a large proportion of the root canal space (*Fig.* 65). However, it is time consuming and, in inexpert hands, dangerous because of the use of red hot instruments. The considerable pressures necessary to condense the gutta percha are unacceptable to some patients as is the thought of a red hot instrument being plunged into their tooth. The access cavity has to be larger than usual and this may weaken the crown.

*d.* GUTTA PERCHA WITH SOLVENTS: Various solvents have been used to render gutta percha more pliable so that it may better conform to the irregular surface of the root canal. Two commonly used solvents are chloroform and eucalyptol. Sometimes instead of using cement an attempt is made to lute gutta percha points to the canal walls with a paste made by dissolving gutta percha in chloroform until a creamy paste is obtained (chloropercha paste).

Gutta percha solvent techniques were first suggested by Callaghan in 1914 and modified by Johnston in 1927. Nygaard-Ostby (1971) advocates the use of Kloroperka N–O which is made by mixing a powder of gutta percha alba, Canada balsam, Colophonium and zinc oxide with chloroform.

There are many advocates of these methods and in expert hands they appear to be as successful as other techniques. However, from first principles they cannot be recommended because the solvents

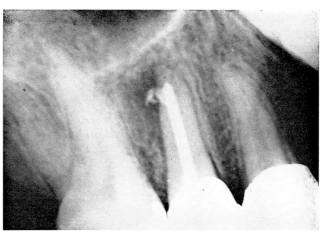

*Fig.* 65. Vertically condensed gutta percha root filling showing three dimensional obturation of canal. Note that the apical foramen is not at the apex of the tooth but, rather, to one side and that this has been occluded with sealer and gutta percha.

are volatile and result in considerable shrinkage of the completed root filling. Further, the solvents are tissue irritants and if accidentally pushed into the periapical tissues may cause considerable irritation and pain.

### 3. *Pastes used alone as Root Filling Materials*

Pastes are normally classified as either resorbable or non-resorbable.

The former normally contain iodoform, do not solidify and are claimed to have antibacterial or germicidal properties. When deposited in the periapical tissues they are quickly removed by macrophage action. 'Kri-I' paste is an example of this type of material and has been discussed on p. 119.

The term 'non-resorbable' is a misnomer, for very few materials are entirely non-resorbable if implanted into the tissues. Even silver cones and steel reamers or files may 'resorb' if implanted in granulomatous tissue (Seltzer, 1971).

'Non-resorbable' pastes (cements) are usually weakly bacteriocidal and set to a resonably hard but porous solid state. If accidentally deposited in the periapical tissue they are removed by phagocytosis much more slowly than the soft resorbable pastes. As seen on p. 117, these pastes and cements usually have a zinc oxide base and are acceptable if used in combination with solid obturating points. Indeed, they must be used with these materials to fill the spaces between the solid cone and the irregular canal walls if a measure of success is to be achieved.

However, what is not acceptable is the use of various pastes and cements for which manufacturers make exorbitant and fallacious claims. These pastes almost invariably contain various toxic medicaments which, apart from being readily resorbable, can be harmful to the tissues. The concept that success can be achieved by the use of drugs alone is, of course, very attractive for it removes the need for tedious and meticulous preparation of the root canal. For this reason some manufacturers offer the profession magical preparations whose use results in 'painless root canal treatment, filling and sealing in one visit' or 'the dressingless method of root canal treatment' or again 'the new effective proven physiological root treatment, by chemical action only, which requires an absolutely minimum of instrumentation' These materials are accompanied by pseudo-scientific explanations and complex formulae, but seldom by any proper histological and clinical investigation results. The use of these materials cannot be recommended.

## CHOICE OF ROOT FILLING TECHNIQUE IN PRACTICE

From the above description of the commonly used techniques in conventional root canal therapy it will be seen that no single technique is applicable to all teeth. The choice of technique will depend on the anatomy of the root canal which is, in turn, influenced by the patient's age, previous dental history and by developmental factors.

To say that any one technique is superior to all others is erroneous and the conscientious practitioner should be conversant with all techniques, evaluate the condition of the tooth requiring treatment and use a technique that will best achieve the principles of successful root therapy, viz. the disinfection of the entire root canal system and the hermetic sealing of the canal from the peridental tissues.

## AFTERCARE AND RECALL

Generally no immediate aftercare is necessary after conventional root canal therapy. However, if sealer has inadvertently been forced through the apical foramen the patient may experience some slight discomfort for a day or two. If this occurs no special treatment is necessary but the patient should be reassured. Very occasionally considerable pain may result after root therapy possibly due to the mechanical or chemical irritation of the periapical tissues. In such circumstances one must ask oneself if the seal at the apex is adequate. If it is, then the periapical reaction will subside without further interference. The use of antibiotics and analgesics may help to overcome this difficult period. If, however, the seal is thought to be inadequate then either the root filling has to be removed to allow adequate drainage or, if this is not possible, apicectomy with retro-filling may offer a solution.

*Recall* is important and the patient should be seen and the tooth X-rayed after six months and one year. Thereafter the patient should be seen at 1- or 2-year intervals for at least a total of 5 years after completion of the treatment.

*The Criteria of Success* are:

1. A clinically symptom-free and functional tooth.

2. The radiographic appearance of the periapical tissues either remains normal (if there was no evidence of bone involvement at the commencement of treatment) or returns to normality by a complete filling of the bony radiolucency.

3. The radiographic appearance of the periodontal ligament appears normal (Harty et al., 1970a).

It would be more correct to examine the radiographic appearance of the lamina dura, for a continuous lamina is proof of normality. However, clinically it is difficult to demonstrate the lamina dura radiographically and it is possible to make it disappear from the X-ray picture by altering the angulation of the tube. Thus, from a practical viewpoint, we look for a continuous radiographic appearance of the periodontal ligament which is easier to see on the X-ray picture (*see* p. 212).

REFERENCES

Bell J. W. (1969) Kri-I paste. *N. Z. Dent. J.* **65**, 96.
Bender I. B. and Seltzer S. (1963) To culture or not to culture? In: Grossman L. I. (ed.), *Transactions of the Third International Conference on Endodontics.* Philadelphia, University of Pennsylvania, p. 83.
Brayton S. M., Davis S. R. and Goldman M. (1973) Gutta-percha root fillings: An in vitro analysis, Part I. *Oral Surg.* **35**, 226.
Callaghan J. R. (1914) Rosin solution for the sealing of dentinal tubuli and as an adjuvant in the filling of root canals. *J. Allied Dent. Soc.* **14**, 53.
Castagnola L. and Orlay H. G. (1952) Treatment of gangrene of the pulp by the Walkhoff method. *Br. Dent. J.* **93**, 93.

Dixon C. M. and Rickert V. G. (1938) Histological verification of results of root canal therapy in experimental animals. *J. Am. Dent. Assoc.* **25**, 1781.

Feldmann G. and Nyborg H. (1962) Tissue reactions to root filling materials. I, Comparison between gutta percha and silver amalgam implanted in rabbit. *Odontol. Revy* **13**, 1.

Friend L. A. and Browne R. M. (1968) Tissue reactions to some root filling materials. *Br. Dent. J.* **125**, 291.

Grieve A. R. and Parkholm J. D. O. (1973) The sealing properties of root filling cements: Further studies. *Br. Dent. J.* **135**, 327.

Grossman L. I. (1958) An improved root canal cement. *J. Am. Dent. Assoc.* **56**, 381.

Grossman L. I. (1974) *Endodontic Practice*, 8th ed. Philadelphia, Lea & Febiger.

Harris W. E. (1971) Disintegration of a silver point: Report of case. *J. Am. Dent. Assoc.* **83**, 868.

Harty F. J., Parkins B. J. and Wengraf A. M. (1970a) Success rate in root canal therapy—A retrospective study of conventional cases. *Br. Dent. J.* **128**, 65.

Harty F. J., Parkins B. J. and Wengraf A. M. (1970b) The success rate of apicectomy—A retrospective study of 1016 cases. *Br. Dent. J.* **129**, 407.

Harty F. J. and Sondoozi A. E. (1972) The status of standardised endodontic instruments. *J. Br. Endodont. Soc.* **6**, 57.

Herd J. R. (1968) Apicoectomy! Why? *Aust. Dent. J.* **13**, 57.

Hess W. and Zurcher E. (1925) *The Anatomy of the Root Canals of the Teeth of the Permanent Dentition and the Anatomy of the Root Canals of the Teeth of the Deciduous Dentition and of the First Permanent Molars.* London, John Bale Sons & Danielsson.

Hill T. R. (1967) An amalgam carrier for use in endodontic treatment. *Dent. Pract. Dent. Rec.* **17**, 285.

Hill T. R. (1970) Root canal therapy by means of apicectomy. *Br. J. Oral Surg.* **7**, 168.

Jasper E. A. (1933) Root canal therapy in modern dentistry. *Dent. Cosmos* **75**, 823.

Kapsimalis P. and Evans R. (1966) Sealing properties of endodontic filling materials using radioactive polar and non-polar isotopes. *Oral Surg.* **22**, 386.

Kawahara H., Yamagami A. and Nakamura M. (1968) Biological testing of dental materials by means of tissue culture. *Int. Dent. J.* **18**, 443.

Keresztesi K. and Kellner G. (1966) The biological effects of root filling materials. *Int. Dent. J.* **16**, 222.

Kramer I. R. H. (1960) The vascular architecture of the human dental pulp. *Archs Oral Biol.* **2**, 177.

Laws A. J. (1964) Kri-I as a root filling paste: Further evidence of its usefulness. *N.Z. Dent. J.* **60**, 180.

Lowman J. V., Burke R. S. and Pelleu G. B. (1973) Patent accessory canals: Incidence in molar furcation region. *Oral Surg.* **36**, 580.

Luks S. (1965) Gutta percha versus silver points in the practice of endodontics. *N.Y. State Dent. J.* **31**, 341.

Marlin J. and Schilder H. (1973) Physical properties of gutta percha when subjected to heat and vertical condensation. *Oral Surg.* **36**, 872.

Marshall F. J. and Massler M. (1961) The sealing of pulpless teeth evaluated with radio-isotopes. *J. Dent. Med.* **16**, 172.

Messing J. J. (1958) Obliteration of the apical third of the root canal with amalgam. *Br. Dent. J.* **104**, 125.

Messing J. J. (1969) Precision apical silver cones. *J. Br. Endodont. Soc.* **3**, 22.

Messing J. J. (1975) Personal communication.

Morse D. R. (1971) The endodontic culture technique: An impractical and unnecessary procedure. *Dent. Clin. North Am.* **15**, 793.

Neagley R. L. (1969) The effect of dowel preparation on the apical seal of endodontically treated teeth. *Oral Surg.* **28**, 739.

Nygaard-Ostby B. (1971) *Introduction to Endodontics.* Oslo, Scandinavian University Books.

Rickert V. G. and Dixon C. M. (1931) The controlling of root surgery. *Proceedings of Eighth International Dental Congress, Paris, 1931.* J. Suppl. Sect. IIIa, Fig. 15.

Rowe A. H. R. (1968) An historical review of materials used for pulp treatment up to the year 1900, Part II. *J. Br. Endodont. Soc.* **2**, 47.

Schilder H. (1967) Filling root canals in three dimensions. *Dent. Clin. North Am.* p. 723.

Schilder H., Goodman A. and Aldrich W. (1974) The thermomechanical properties of gutta percha. I, The compressibility of gutta percha. *Oral Surg.* **37**, 946.

Schroeder A. (1957) Zum Problem der Bakteriedichten Wurzelkanal Versorgung. *Zahnærztl. Welt.* **58**, 531.

Seltzer S., Bender I. B. and Turkenkopf S. (1963) Factors affecting successful repair after root canal therapy. *J. Am. Dent. Assoc.* **67**, 651.

Seltzer S., Soltanoff W. and Bender I. B. (1969) Epithelial proliferation in periapical lesions. *Oral Surg.* **27**, 111.

Seltzer S. (1971) *Endodontology: Biologic Considerations in Endodontic Procedures.* New York, McGraw-Hill.

Talim S. T. and Singh I. (1967) Sealing of root canal fillings in 'vivo' conditions as assessed by radioactive iodine. *J. Indian Dent. Ass.* **39**, 198.

# CHAPTER 8

# SURGICAL ENDODONTICS

THE relief of pain following incision and drainage of a swelling of dental origin was known to the Egyptians as early as the third millennium B.C. Indeed mandibles exist with bur holes which experts consider could only have been made *in vivo* for the relief of pain due to an alveolar abscess (Hill, 1970). Transplantation and re-implantation appears to be the only other surgical technique practised until the middle of the nineteenth century.

In 1884 Farrar, in a paper entitled 'Radical and Heroic Treatment of Alveolar Abscess by Amputation of Roots of Teeth with a Description and Application of the Cantilever Crown', advocated an apicectomy technique which was truly radical and certainly heroic. This was not an entirely successful technique because the concept of seal at the apex was not understood and also because the foreshortening of the root made post-retained tooth restoration difficult.

Surgical endodontics, until relatively recently, was considered to be synonymous with apicectomy. Nowadays the term 'surgical endodontics' includes the following operations under which the subject will be discussed:

1. Incision and drainage of soft tissue swellings.
2. Surgical fistulation.
3. Periapical curettage.
4. Apicectomy.
5. Root amputation.
6. Replantation and transplantation.
7. Endodontic endosseous stabilization.

In the field of general surgery surgical endodontics is classified as a relatively minor procedure. Nevertheless the contra-indications applying to general surgery apply equally well to endodontic surgery which should never be carried out if alternative conventional root canal therapy techniques are possible.

## 1. INCISION AND DRAINAGE

With the advent of the antibiotics some dental surgeons are abandoning the time honoured precept that 'the sun should never set on undrained pus' and treat endodontic emergencies by chemotherapy alone. This is to be deplored, for the emergency treatment for a tooth with a periapical abscess is still drainage. The use of antibiotics is not an alternative treatment and whilst it may contain the infection in time it does not relieve the patient of his acute symptoms immediately. On the other hand, drainage of an acute swelling either through the tooth or through the soft tissues provides almost instantaneous relief.

Wherever possible the canal should be emptied and cleaned so that unimpeded drainage can take place. If drainage does not occur, or if the root canal cannot be negotiated, the patient should be instructed to use frequent hot mouth baths to encourage pointing. If and when there is a fluctuant swelling incision and drainage through the mucosa is essential.

Where drainage either through the tooth or through the mucosa is unobtainable then antibiotics should be prescribed to contain the infection during the acute stage.

In such cases local analgesia is difficult if not impossible and in any event a local analgesic should not be injected into inflamed tissues. Topical analgesics are useful and applied copiously to the area to be incised on a swab or cottonwool ball. It is imperative that sufficient time be allowed for the analgesic to work and five minutes should be the minimum.

A 'refrigeration' analgesia is sometimes useful and this is achieved by spraying the tissue with a volatile material such as ethyl chloride until a white frost appears in the area to be incised. This material must be used carefully for it is a potent general anaesthetic and the back of the throat must be protected with a gauze pack to prevent loss of consciousness (Roberts and Sowray, 1970). The eyes must also be protected against injury from the spray.

The incision should be made when it is reasonably certain that pus is present and should be directed at the centre of the most fluctuant area of the swelling. The incision is made with a sharp No. 15 Bard Parker blade in a mesiodistal direction. An alternative method of obtaining drainage is described on p. 14. Squeezing the abscess before or after incision should be avoided as it may cause pus to invade fresh tissue. The patient should be instructed to use frequent warm saline mouth washes to irrigate the area and 'disinfect' the mouth generally. The use of drainage tubes or rubber dam to keep the wound open and promote drainage is not usually necessary.

The administration of antibiotics in routine endodontic practice is seldom necessary and, as has been mentioned before, the use of antibiotics is not an alternative for adequate drainage. However, if the dental infection is severe enough to cause general malaise with raised temperature, or if the infection appears to be general rather than localized or if the patient's general medical history requires it, then supportive antibiotic treatment should be instituted at once (*see* p. 14).

## 2. SURGICAL FISTULATION

The term 'fistulation' is not strictly correct for a fistula is a patho-
logic communication between a cavity lined with epithelium and
the oral mucosa whilst a 'sinus' is a tract between a suppurating
area and the oral mucosa.

A tooth with a sinus is usually painless and for this reason routine
fistulation (sinus formation) is advocated by some practitioners.

This procedure is not often necessary because drainage and
thorough débridement of the root canal is usually sufficient to overcome immediate symptoms or prevent an acute exacerbation.
On the very rare occasion when drainage and débridement is not
possible then the alternative rests between the control of infection
and pain with antibiotics and with analgesics and surgical fistulation. This is carried out under local or general anaesthesia when a
small incision is made over the apex of the involved tooth. The lips
of the wound are opened slightly to permit the insertion of a small
round bur which is advanced until the cortical plate is punctured,
thus allowing drainage. In practice it is not easy to make this
penetration accurately over the apex.

## 3. PERIAPICAL CURETTAGE

Periapical curettage is defined as the operation in which diseased
periapical tissue is removed surgically following root filling, the root
apex being left in position. Sometimes the cemental surface of the
root apex is curetted (British Standards Institution, 1969).

This operation was considered essential following the root filling
of any tooth. It is now performed very rarely because of the realization that it contributes nothing to the ultimate success of the root
filling. The root filling must stand or fall by the efficacy of its seal.
If the seal is adequate the periapical tissue will heal without further
interference. If the seal is inadequate then either the root filling
must be replaced conventionally or the apex sealed with a retrograde amalgam, which implies the removal of portion of the root and
it is then an apicectomy rather than an apical curettage.

Thus both the term and the practice of apical curettage are
deprecated.

## 4. APICECTOMY

An apicectomy is defined as the operation of removing the root
apex, usually with surrounding tissue, the root canal being filled
either before or immediately after the removal of the root apex.
Alternative terms are 'root resection' and 'root amputation' both of
which are deprecated (British Standards Institution, 1969). The
object of the operation is to obtain an apical seal where this cannot
be achieved by conventional root canal therapy.

## Indications

a. In cases of extreme apical curvature, dilaceration or where there is a calcific barrier in the pulp cavity.

b. Where the apex is open thus preventing the placement of an adequate seal conventionally.

c. In teeth with lateral canals or perforations which are accessible for filling at operation.

d. In already crowned teeth where the coronal approach is blocked by a post which cannot be removed.

e. Teeth in which a fractured instrument requires removal but cannot be removed in any other way.

f. Fracture of the apical third of the root where the apex requires removal.

g. Where cystic degeneration of a granuloma is suspected. This is in fact surprisingly rare and X-rays may be very misleading.

h. Expediency—if the patient has insufficient time for root canal therapy.

i. To remove a foreign body, such as excess root canal sealer, from the periapical tissues. (A reamer broken at the apex will on occasions prove to be an adequate root filling, and should only be removed if found to be an inadequate seal.)

## Contra-indications

a. Medical

1. In the presence of acute infection.

2. In patients with debilitating disease, such as uncontrolled diabetes or nephritis, which may retard healing and which may increase the risk of secondary infection.

3. Haemophilia and other haemorrhagic diseases such as Christmas disease, purpura, von Willebrand's disease and in severe liver dysfunction which may often lead to bleeding tendencies.

4. In patients on anticoagulant therapy because of the increased risk of excessive haemorrhage.

5. In patients on steroid therapy. Patients whose dosage of adrenocortical steroid has been high and of long duration may develop some degree of degeneration of the adrenal

144

cortex. Because of this the patient's protective mechanism against stress is unable to function properly and this renders him liable to attacks of faintness, nausea, vomiting, and to hypotension which may prove fatal. It is possible to treat patients on steroid therapy, but the patient's physician should be consulted, and he may be able to advise on temporary increase in the dose of steroid in order to counteract the effects of stress. It is as well to remember that they may not recover from adrenocortical insufficiency for up to 2 years.

6. Normally, apicectomy is carried out under local analgesia, and a vasoconstrictor is necessary to produce a degree of vasoconstriction which facilitates the operation. Certain patients, e.g. patients with myocardial ischaemia, may have an attack of angina pectoris if adrenaline is one of the constituents of the analgesic solution.

7. Extremely nervous and emotional patients and patients with hyperthyroidism. Because of the lack of co-operation these patients may have to be treated under general anaesthesia.

8. Pregnant women, as far as possible, should be treated during the middle trimester.

9. In the presence of local vascular abnormalities such as a haemangioma.

In all the above situations it may be possible to treat the patient by apicectomy, but this should not be done without consulting the patient's physician.

## b. Local

1. If surrounding tissues are likely to be damaged because of the operation (e.g. inferior dental nerve, maxillary sinus, apices of other teeth).

2. Where the root length is such that further root removal will shorten the root to such a degree that permanent restoration of the tooth becomes impossible.

### Method and Rationale

As in conventional root canal therapy the object of the treatment is to seal the apical foramen.

*Instruments for Apicectomy*

An apicectomy kit may be prepared from instruments chosen
from the following:

Cartridge syringe
Mouth mirror No. 4
Probes, right angle No. 6
    sickle No. 54
    Briault No. 11
Tweezers, 'College pattern' No. 8
Scalpel with No. 15 Bard-Parker blade
Periosteal elevator No. 1 or No. 9
Osteo-Mitchell trimmer No. 4
Cement spatula
Enamel chisel No. 84
Excavators Nos. 72/73
            125/126
            206/207
            212/213
            G5
            G6
Plastic instruments Nos. 155  (Hobson)
                    156  (Hobson)
                     49  (Baldwin)
                  154
                  154S
Hunts' Water Syringe (or 10 ml disposable syringe with specially adapted
    metal nozzle)
Metal mug
Sucker head tips (with length of stainless-steel wire for clearing blockages)
Porcelain dish containing the following burs:
    Straight—Round No. 2 (010) and 5 (016)
           —Tapered fissure No. 701 (012) and 702 (016)
    Right angle—Round No. $\frac{1}{4}$ (005) and $\frac{1}{2}$ (006)
Hill Endodontic Amalgam Carrier
Austin retractor
Needle holder
Spencer-Wells forceps
Tissue forceps (Gillies or McIndoe dissection forceps—1 × 2 teeth)
Small scissors
Aluminium disposable dish or stainless-steel kidney dish (for waste)
Gauze swabs

All of the above should be placed in a metal box and sterilized
by autoclaving, prior to operation.

The following are also necessary and are now normally available
in sterile packs:

Scalpel and scalpel blades
Saline
Bone wax W 810
Siliconized black silk suture on 19 mm $\frac{3}{8}$ circle needle

*Anaesthesia*

The operation is usually carried out under local analgesia with an
analgesic containing adrenaline in order to control haemorrhage.
The analgesia must be adequate. For example, an upper lateral
incisor will require buccal infiltration on *both* sides of the midline

146

and a palatal infiltration distal to the tooth to anaesthetize the greater palatine nerve, and will also require an infiltration directed into the incisive papilla to block the long sphenopalatine nerve (Roberts and Sowray, 1970).

If a general anaesthetic is used then, with the anaesthetists' permission, a local analgesic containing adrenaline should be injected because it facilitates the operation by reducing haemorrhage and thus improving visibility.

*Incision*

Access to the apical area is obtained by raising a flap of muco-periosteum, either through the labial or buccal mucosa or by raising a gingival flap. In either event the reflected tissue must be of sufficient area to give good vision and access to the periapical area. It should include both mucosa and periosteum, thus opening one tissue plane only. When replaced the suture line should be on sound bone.

MUCOSAL INCISION: This can be either straight or convex towards the crown. It should be long enough to give adequate access and extend down to bone. There is no virtue in inadequate visibility and poor access. The incision should include one tooth on either side and often more but it should not normally encroach on the reflection of the mucosa nor lie over the bony lesion itself. This will ensure that the final suture line lies on sound bone. On the other hand, the incision should not be so close to the gingival margin as to endanger the blood supply of the papillae. If the incision has to lie closer than 5 mm from the gingival margin (for example, when a labial root perforation has to be filled) then the inverse bevel gingival incision should be considered. In the case of upper central incisors the incision should try to avoid the fraenum, but if this is not possible the fraenum is cut through cleanly and sutured. A large fraenum may be conveniently reduced in size during this operation.

The advantages of the mucosal incision are that if healing does not occur by first intention the resultant scar will not show. It is also easier to carry out than the gingival incision which requires more than average skill if the gingival margin is not to be damaged.

INVERSE BEVEL GINGIVAL INCISION: This has been suggested by Hill (1974) as being 'superior to other designs with regard to healing and lack of scar formation'. It is extremely useful in the lower anterior region where the raising of the mucoperiosteal flap over the labial portion of the mandible gives good access and, more import-antly, allows good vision and identification of bony landmarks, thus making it relatively easy to find the apex of a particular tooth. It is also useful when raising a flap around crowned teeth for it is possible to reposition the flap gingivally with greater precision and without any undue strain from sutures.

The technique, as described by Hill, is similar to the standard gingival line approach used for many years, and entails the lifting of the attached mucoperiosteum from the gingival crevice of the teeth. Relieving incisions are made and these extend into the buccal sulcus so that the flap includes the interdental papilla at each end.

In the inverse bevel modification (*Fig.* 66) the papilla is split by the relieving incision so that the circular fibres of the periodontium and the gingival crevices are maintained on the teeth on either side of the flap. The raised flap then consists of the gingival crevice

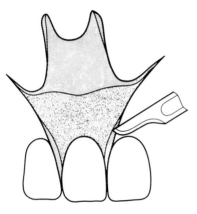

*Fig.* 66. Modification of the gingival line incision showing the splitting of the papilla.(*Photograph by courtesy of Mr. T. R. Hill.*)

and the bulk of the papilla of the teeth in question. This is achieved by angulating the scalpel blade away from the gingival crevice of the neighbouring teeth in the region of the interdental papilla. The remainder of the relieving incision goes straight through the mucosa and periosteum.

*Flap Reflection*

Flap reflection is carried out with a stout edged periosteal elevator. The instrument should be pressed firmly to bone and the periosteum and mucosa reflected without tearing. The same instrument is then used as a retractor. It is also possible to use, in the maxilla, a specially designed retractor which has the advantage of freeing the hand otherwise holding the retractor (Hill, 1974) (*Fig.* 67).

The flap should not be subjected to excessive movement otherwise bleeding will obscure unduly the operative field.

*The Bony Window*

It is necessary to remove sufficient of the outer alveolar plate to see the periapical region clearly. Location of this region is easy if the area of bone loss is large and there is already a perforation of the bone. Conversely, where the periapical bone loss is minimal, it can be difficult to locate the apex, and the following points may help.

1. Anatomical landmarks on the bone (e.g. the ridge formed by a canine) are helpful.

2. From the X-ray of the root being sought the relationship to the neighbouring teeth may be seen.

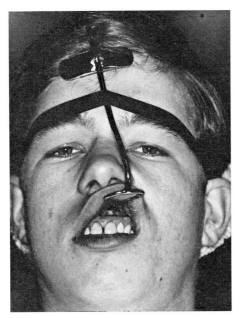

*Fig.* 67. Hill flap retractor which has the advantage of freeing the hand normally holding the retractor.

3. A wire placed in the root canal shows its direction and therefore the probable site of the apex.

4. Where it is possible to calculate the tooth length from a diagnostic wire X-ray, this length may be marked on the bone so as to pinpoint the position of the apex (*Fig.* 68).

5. The apex of a maxillary lateral incisor is usually deeply placed towards the palatal.

6. If there is no visible perforation, probing the bone with a sharp probe will often reveal a small hole in the cortical bone, which is nearly always eroded where there is an area of rarefaction on the X-ray (Wengraf, 1964).

149

If there is only a thin layer of bone over the apex, it is easily removed by paring with an excavator or a chisel using finger pressure. Alternatively a round bur may be used, working from the centre to the periphery.

If there is no periapical bony lesion or the area is small or deep, a bony window has to be cut to reach the apex. Once the site of the apex has been carefully determined, the shape of the bony window may be outlined by making a series of bur holes with a No. 3 (I.S.O.

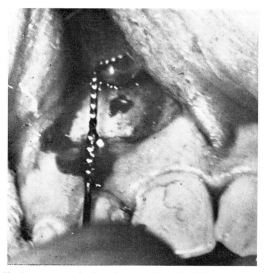

*Fig.* 68. Reamer marked to show the length of the root canal and used to identify the site of the root apex.

No. 012) round bur, extending to just below the alveolar plate. (If a fissure bur is used for this stage, it must *not* penetrate deeply below the alveolar plate, or the root may be partly severed at the wrong level.) While cutting bone with a bur, the site should be irrigated continuously with normal saline, which prevents the clogging of the bur and this, in turn, prevents the generation of heat which may lead to bone necrosis.

*Débridement*

Once the outer plate has been removed, the periapical cavity should be cleaned with excavators so as to expose the root apex. Over-enthusiastic curettage should be avoided at this stage for it will cause the wound to bleed which may make apex identification difficult. The apex can then be examined and the correct level for resection determined.

*Resection*

The amount of root that has to be resected will depend on the type of root filling required. Ideally the root should be planed back until the root filling (if present) is just exposed and seen to occlude the apex. If no root filling is present the canal should be identified and sufficient root apex removed to allow for the preparation of an undercut Class I type cavity. Formerly it was thought that the root had to be resected to the base of the bony cavity surrounding the apex. This is no longer considered correct practice for two reasons. Firstly shortening a root surgically decreases the available root length for a subsequent post crown and also decreases the intra-alveolar lever arm thereby worsening or exaggerating the effects of occlusal trauma (Stallard, 1973). Secondly, excessive root resection contradicts the principles of root therapy, i.e. to place a hermetic seal as close to the apex of a tooth as possible and allow the tooth to remain in function within the dental arch. If the seal at the apex is adequate then resolution of the periapical area will occur irrespective of where the new mechanically created apex is placed.

When the level of root resection is determined the root apex is removed by slicing through the root with a 701 or 702 tapered fissure bur (I.S.O. No. 012 or 016). The use of a flat fissure bur is not recommended because it may jam in the root and fracture. Cutting is, of course, carried out under a stream of sterile water or saline so that visibility is improved and no debris falls within the surrounding bony cavity.

The angle at which the root is resected is important and depends on the type of root filling present or, if the canal is unfilled, on the type of root filling that will be inserted after resection (*see below*).

*Sealing the Apex*

Controversy exists on whether the root filling should be placed before or after resection. Some researchers consider that better results were obtained when the root filling was placed before surgery (Tschamer, 1955; Harnisch and Grieger, 1967) whilst others (Mattila and Altonen, 1968; Nordenram and Svärdström, 1970; Rud and Andreasen, 1972) considered that in all cases the apex should be resected first, the canal débrided and filled at operation.

The feeling at the Institute of Dental Surgery is that both viewpoints have merit but where possible the canal should be prepared and filled prior to resection because it is easier to dry the canal as there is no bleeding from the periapical tissues. It is also considered that for all apicectomy techniques the root filling of choice is amalgam because this gives a three dimensional, well condensed root filling that sets hard and can not be disturbed during resection.

151

A further advantage is that a mechanical stop can be cut in the root canal against which amalgam is condensed and this stop prevents the accidental extrusion of the root filling during subsequent fabrication and insertion of a post-retained crown. (*See below.*)

Gutta percha or silver points are not used because the former may be softened and pulled away from the sides of the canal by the bur during the resection of the apex. A silver point cemented with sealer is often partly or completely loosened by the vibration of the bur as it is cut through during the resection.

Because apicected teeth are likely to need a post-retained crown the ideal filling material should occlude only the apical 3 mm of canal after resection and, as mentioned above, it should be sufficiently retentive so as not to be dislodged either at apicectomy or during the subsequent preparation or insertion of a post-retained restoration.

### Apicectomy Sealing Techniques

The apex may be sealed by one of three methods, viz.: (1) The conventional; (2) The retrograde; (3) The through-and-through.

### 1. *The Conventional Method* (*Fig.* 69)

This method is used when the greater portion of the root canal can be negotiated through the usual access cavity into the pulp chamber, but where the apical region of the canal is not readily accessible. The root seal is placed as near to the apex as possible and the root is then resected to the level of this seal.

TECHNIQUE

1. An access cavity in line with the greater portion of root canal is made through the palatal, lingual or occlusal surface of the tooth.

2. A diagnostic X-ray of the tooth is taken using a stout straight diagnostic wire or reamer which is passed as far apically as possible without undue bending. The depth of penetration is marked on the diagnostic wire or reamer and this length noted because it gives a good indication, at operation, of the site of the apex.

3. The tooth is now reamed to this level until fresh dentine is removed from the apical region of the root canal.

4. Further reaming is continued using 2 or 3 larger sizes of reamer at a level 2 or 3 mm coronally from the initial reaming. This provides a step within the root canal which prevents the apical seal from being dislodged apically during a subsequent post-retained crown preparation.

5. A file is used to clean any areas of the root canal not reached by the reamers.

6. Amalgam is triturated normally but excess mercury is not squeezed out. It is introduced into the root canal, in small increments, by means of one of the special amalgam carriers, developed by Messing* (1958) or by Hill† (1964). A mark should be made on the carrier to indicate the depth of the prepared canal. Each increment is condensed with a flat-ended fine plugger of suitable diameter, which is marked in the same way as the carrier. (These pluggers are easily made from stainless-steel orthodontic wire of suitable diameter.)

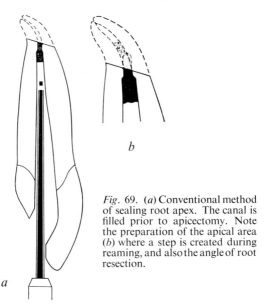

*b*

*a*

Fig. 69. (*a*) Conventional method of sealing root apex. The canal is filled prior to apicectomy. Note the preparation of the apical area (*b*) where a step is created during reaming, and also the angle of root resection.

Ideally, the amalgam should be packed into a dry canal. If, however, the canal is wet due to apical seapage the first increment of amalgam will be contaminated with moisture, but will be an effective barrier to further leakage. The canal is then re-dried and the amalgam condensation continued until 3–4 mm of the apical portion of the canal is filled. (The contaminated amalgam is later removed during the surgical procedure.)

7. The remainder of the canal is left empty and the access cavity sealed with a suitable filling material.

*Messing Endodontic Gun: Produits Dentaires, Vevey, Switzerland.
†Hill Endodontic Amalgam Carrier: P. J. Clark & Co. Ltd., 1–6 Speedy Place, Cromer Street, London WC1H 8BX.

8. The apex is then resected surgically as described on p. 151. The angle of resection should be such that the resected root face should be clearly visible and a visual check can be made to ascertain that the root filling is surrounded by sound dentine. The efficiency of the seal should be tested with a probe and if found to be defective then a retrograde root filling should be placed as well (*see below*). This is a simple matter for the existing amalgam root filling forms a base against which fresh amalgam can be condensed.

The root resection is carried out under a stream of sterile water or saline to improve visibility and prevent debris from lodging in the bony cavity. It also has the added advantage of indicating when the bur has begun to cut the amalgam as evidenced by the stained slurry at the site of resection. Whilst the deposition of amalgam particles is, of itself, not harmful it may result in an amalgam tattoo of the mucosa and in any event looks 'untidy' on a radiograph. This can be prevented by packing the bony cavity with the tail of a swab dampened in sterile water or saline. Alternatively the entire cavity can be packed with bone wax* and the wax overlying the root apex trimmed back prior to resection and amalgam placement. This technique has the added advantage of controlling the bleeding and thus giving a dry field of operation. When the root filling has been completed the bone wax with any trapped debris is carefully removed, and the site irrigated with saline (Rothschild, 1970; Selden, 1970).

The flaps are re-apposed and sutured as described on p. 157. It is important that the flap is not sutured whilst there is bony bleeding of any consequence for this will allow blood to be trapped under the soft tissues and cause an unsightly ecchymosis.

2. *The Retrograde Method* (*Fig.* 70)
This method is indicated where an apical seal has to be placed directly into the apical portion of a root canal that is inaccessible through the conventional approach (e.g. in a dilacerated tooth or in a tooth with an adequate post crown which cannot be removed easily.)

TECHNIQUE

1. Analgesia, flap reflection, and access to the apex are carried out as described on pp. 146–148.

2. The apex of the tooth is located and resected *at an angle of about 45°* to the long axis of the tooth so that the root face and canal orifice are clearly visible to the operator. A small cavity is then cut into this root face incorporating the canal

---

*Ethicon Bone Wax W 810: Ethicon Ltd., Bankhead Avenue, Edinburgh EH11 4HE.

orifice. This is best carried out with a size $\frac{1}{4}$ or $\frac{1}{2}$ (I.S.O.
No. 005 or 006) round bur in a right angled handpiece.
Adequate undercuts are prepared in the mesial, distal and
palatal or lingual and if possible the labial wall of the cavity
Whilst special sub-miniature endodontic hand pieces are
available for the preparation of the apical cavity they are not
essential and a conventional handpiece is adequate.

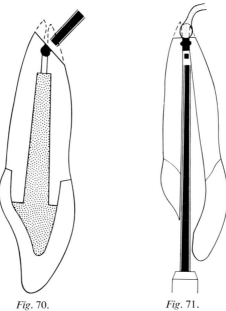

*Fig*. 70.                    *Fig*. 71.

*Fig*. 70. The retrograde method. Note that the apex is resected at
an angle of 45° to the long axis of the tooth so that the amputated
root face and root canal orifice are clearly visible.

*Fig*. 71. The through-and-through method. In this instance apex
resection should be at right angles to the long axis of the tooth.

3. Amalgam is prepared in the usual way and small increments
   introduced into the dried cavity by means of an endodontic
   amalgam carrier. Each increment is condensed with a suitable
   plastic instrument or fine amalgam plugger.

   As before the bony cavity may be packed off with ribbon
   gauze or bone wax. However, the use of the Messing or Hill
   gun makes the accidental deposition of amalgam in the
   peridental area rare because the fine diameter of the instrument tip makes it easy to deposit the amalgam inside the
   prepared apical cavity. Any excess during condensation is
   easily seen and removed with an excavator as it occurs.

155

4. When the apical cavity is filled satisfactorily (the condensation should be as good as one would expect of a well condensed Class I cavity elsewhere in the mouth), the ribbon gauze or bone wax packing is removed, the periapical area is examined carefully for excess amalgam, and if necessary X-rayed to help in the identification and removal of the amalgam debris, irrigated and the flap re-apposed and sutured as described on p. 157.

### 3. The 'Through-and-Through' Method (*Fig. 71*)

This is a combination of the two preceding methods and is used in cases where the apical foramen is open and has an inadequate constriction against which to pack amalgam.

TECHNIQUE:

1. Analgesia, flap retraction and access to the apex are carried out as described on pp. 146–148.

2. The root canal is reamed and filed until fresh dentine is exposed.

3. The apex of the tooth is then resected to produce a flat surface *at right angles* to the root canal. Undercuts are prepared with a size $\frac{1}{2}$ or $\frac{1}{4}$ (I.S.O. No. 005 or 006) round bur about 1·5 mm from the resected root end. It is generally only possible to place undercuts mesially, distally, and palatally or lingually, and these are sufficient to anchor the filling so that it will not be dislodged during post crown preparation.

4. The amalgam root seal can be placed in either of two ways.
    a. The apical end is occluded with a suitable instrument such as a ball-ended burnisher whose diameter is large enough to occlude the apical foramen. Amalgam is then packed through the coronal access cavity with an endodontic amalgam carrier and condensed from that end, against the apical instrument stop, in the same manner as for the conventional method. Again 2–3 mm of amalgam root filling are sufficient.
    b. A piece of stout wire or a silver point whose blunt end is of sufficient diameter to jam some 2–3 mm from the resected end is placed in the canal through the access cavity and held in position with a gutta percha plug. If a silver point is used the tapering end can be bent against the incisal or occlusal surface of the tooth thus helping to stabilize the point within the root canal. Amalgam is then packed into the canal as in the retrograde method until the apical 2–3 mm are completely occluded with a well condensed

filling. The precautions against dropping amalgam particles in the bony cavity are the same as for the retrograde method.

At the completion of the filling the silver point of wire stop is removed from the canal, the bony cavity cleared of ribbon gauze or bone wax packing, checked for amalgam contamination, and irrigated. When haemorrhage has ceased the flap is repositioned and sutured as discussed below.

*Wound Closure*

At the completion of the operation and irrespective of the type of incision, the flap design and the root filling technique used, the bony cavity is re-examined for root filling contamination and any residual granulation tissue curetted. Controversy exists about the necessity of periapical curettage. Some authorities consider that this is not necessary for the granulation tissue is not normally invaded by bacteria. Others consider that granulation tissue often contains epithelium which may develop into a radicular cyst if stimulated by re-infection of the root canal. It is also possible that the epithelium will form a cover over the root surface which may prevent repair into a normal periodontal space (Andreasen and Rud, 1972). This situation may be present in cases where an apicectomy is successful clinically but where the radiographic picture continues to show a thickened periodontal ligament rather than a normal periodontal space with a 'clean' lamina dura.

As mentioned before the wound should not be sutured until haemorrhage has ceased so that the blood clot trapped beneath the flap is of minimal size, thus preventing an ecchymosis due to blood extravasation and breakdown of the clot. Bruising does occur in about 5 per cent of cases and if severe may involve the mandible and the neck regardless of the site of operation. This is possibly due to the drainage of the area. If bleeding is excessive a small rectangular-shaped drain can be cut from a sheet of rubber dam, folded in half lengthwise and attached with a single suture so that oozing of the wound continues without an excessive build up of pressure below the apposed flap. Such a drain should be removed in 24 hours.

The lips of the wound are re-apposed and sutured with interrupted black siliconized silk sutures crossing the wound at right angles. An eyeless $\frac{3}{8}$ circle 19 mm atraumatic needle with 4·0* silk is particularly useful as there is only one strand of very fine silk. The number of sutures necessary is difficult to define but the general rule is that they should not be placed closer to each other than necessary and the wound edges should neither overlap or show a depression.

---

*Davis & Geck—Cyanamid of G.B. Limited, Bush House, Aldwych, London WC2 B4PU.

*Aftercare*

Analgesics should be prescribed for postoperative pain and the patient should be warned that there may be some postoperative oedema and bruising. The patient should spend a quiet day after the operation, a thing which he or she will, in any case, wish to do. On the following day, the patient should be advised to clean the teeth normally except for the affected area, which may be swabbed with cottonwool and water or a mild antiseptic. Excessive lip movements, and inspection of the suture line should be discouraged. Warm saline mouth washes provide some relief. The patient should be advised to return in the event of haemorrhage or excess swelling. Persistent haemorrhage is not common. To treat it, the sutures are removed and the cavity packed with fibrin foam and re-sutured. Sutures are routinely removed after 3–5 days, but in the lower anterior region 7 days may be preferable as the tissue is more friable than in the maxilla.

*Recall*

The patient should be seen and the tooth investigated and X-rayed after 6 months and 1 year. Thereafter the patient should be seen at 1- or 2-year intervals for at least 5 years after the completion of the treatment.

Success in apicectomy, and indeed in conventional root canal therapy, is difficult to define for it depends on the observer's viewpoint. A tooth which is symptomless and gives rise to no complaints by the patient may be considered, by some, to be successfully treated without recourse to postoperative radiography. On the other hand, many will undertake conventional root therapy with or without apicectomy on the strength of a radiograph showing evidence of apical rarefaction and thus success must take into account the final radiographic picture some time after treatment.

The following criteria have been suggested (Harty et al., 1970):

1. The tooth remains clinically symptomless and functional for 2 or more years, at which time there should be an absence of—
   *a.* Tenderness
   *b.* Persistent sinus.
   *c.* Breakdown of incision
   *d.* Recurrence of swelling
   *e.* Tenderness, discomfort or pain over the operation site
   *f.* Excess mobility of the tooth
   *g.* Drifting of the tooth because of lack of bony support or inadequate root length
   *h.* Periodontal disease of iatrogenic origin.

2. The radiographic appearance of the periodontal ligament remains normal or returns to normality.
3. There is no radiological evidence of any abnormality.

These criteria apply to both conventional root canal therapy and apicectomy. However, the radiographic interpretation of success is more difficult in apicectomy for, where a large bony cavity is present, as often it is before and must be immediately after treatment, the repair by connective tissue alone is more common than in conventional root canal therapy. Thus, if a radiolucent apical area remains, the case cannot be regarded as successful unless this area is clearly separated from the amputated root and the radiographic appearance of the periodontal ligament is normal (*Fig.* 72).

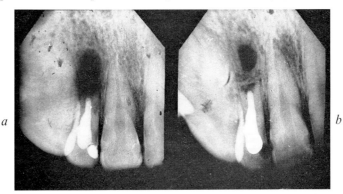

*a*  *b*

*Fig.* 72. *a,* Radiograph immediately postoperatively. *b,* Radiograph 18 months later showing bone deposition periapically and a residual radiolucent area at a distance from the amputated apex.

These residual radiolucent apical areas are relatively common and result from irreversible damage, by infection or during operation, of either or both the outer or inner cortical plate (Wengraf, 1964). It is often argued that in the presence of such irreversible bony destruction the case can never be considered successful. However, in such cases the radiolucency can be accepted provided the periodontal ligament is seen to be radiographically continuous and of normal thickness.

*Repair of Perforations and the Filling of*
*Accessory and Lateral Canals by Surgical Means*

By definition the repair of perforations and lateral canals is not an apicectomy. However, for convenience they are considered under this section because the surgical approach and the obliteration of the perforation or of the orifice of the accessory canal are identical to the apicectomy operation.

1. *Accessory Canals* occur in about 25 per cent of teeth. They are usually located in the apical third of the tooth and their débridement and filling is almost impossible because they usually lie at right angles to the main canal. It may be possible to clean them by using chlorinated soda solution and it is claimed that lateral or vertical condensation techniques afford the best way of sealing these canals, because the condensation of the gutta percha forces the sealer into the canal and this sealer forms a satisfactory root filling.

Clinically, the inadequate filling of accessory canals is the cause of a surprisingly small number of failures. Ingle (1965) suggests that this is because the tissue in lateral canals remains vital even though the contents of the main canal are necrotic. He considers that the lateral canal may have its own blood supply from vessels in the periodontal ligament and is thus independent of the blood supply of the main canal.

Generally accessory canals are not a problem for the above reason and also because they occur in the apical third of the root thus making them short in length, likely to be filled satisfactorily at their junction with the main canal and also because their openings into the periodontal space may be obliterated by cementum which is normally deposited in this area of the root. If they create a problem, where possible, an apicectomy type operation with retrograde amalgam filling is usually successful.

Occasionally, accessory canals may be labial or palatal in direction, and are thus not visible on X-ray due to the superimposition of the main canal. These canals are impossible to detect and are an occasional source of unexplained failure of root canal therapy.

2. *Lateral Canals* frequently occur in the furcation areas of multi-rooted teeth and sometimes in the middle and coronal thirds of the root. Canals in the furcation areas are difficult to deal with and are best approached and filled through the pulp chamber (*see Fig.* 63, p. 131).

Those in the middle or coronal third of the root, if readily accessible, i.e. on the buccal root surfaces, are demonstrated by raising an inverse bevel gingival flap and examining the bone and root surface for a fault. When the canal orifice is found a small amount of bone is removed with either a chisel, an excavator, or with a slowly rotating round bur and the smallest possible Class I type cavity prepared in the root. Undercuts are formed in the wall as for a retrograde apicectomy and the cavity is filled with amalgam.

It is important that the least possible amount of bone be removed and that the filling surface be kept as small as possible because once the cementum has been removed from the root face the periodontal tissue will not reattach on the denuded root.

3. *Perforations* are usually caused by a bur or engine reamer and are thus amenable, due to their direction, to further instrumentation. The false canal and foramen (perforation) should be sealed in the same manner as the natural root canal with sealer and gutta percha, or sealer alone, either at the same time as the main canal or before it. If they are coronally placed, the periodontal aspect of the perforation is plugged from within with a sheet of gold foil and this is backed up and held in place by amalgam (Leggett, 1975).

If the perforation presents a large surface to the periodontal tissues and is the cause of an area of bone resorption, a better seal can be achieved by uncovering the perforation by a surgical approach, cutting retention in the cavity, and filling with amalgam as described above.

Perforations caused by either internal or external resorption, if favourable from an anatomical viewpoint and of moderate size can be repaired in the same manner.

## 5. ROOT AMPUTATION

Root amputation is defined as the operation of removing an entire root of a multi-rooted tooth, which has been root filled, because of technical difficulty in the treatment of this root, in order to facilitate cleaning of the tissues in the region of the roots (BS 4492: 1969).

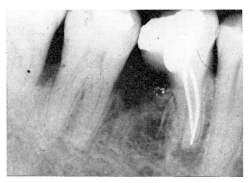

*Fig.* 73. Amputation of the distal root of the mandibular first molar. The crown is left intact and the tissue surface is re-shaped to a self cleansing form.

The term 'root resection' should not be used because it is often used as a synonym for apicectomy and may lead to confusion. Root amputation (*Fig.* 73) implies that the crown is left intact, but in practice it is generally re-shaped to a self-cleansing form. 'Hemi-section' refers to the division of the tooth in half and the removal of the diseased portion with attached root or roots. The division is made bucco-lingually in two rooted mandibular molars and mesio-distally in maxillary molars and premolars. Root amputation or hemisection is generally necessary for periodontal reasons (*Fig.* 74) but is also useful in teeth with extensive carious lesions which extend subgingivally in one area of the root and where it is not possible to place an adequate restoration (*see* Chapter 10).

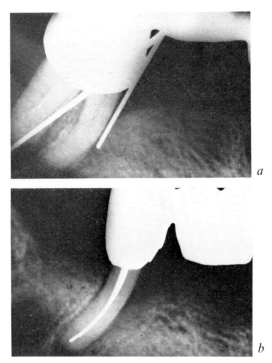

*a*

*b*

*Fig.* 74. *a*, Lower second molar with gross periodontal involvement of distal root as evidenced by the silver point marker placed in the periodontal pocket. *b*, Tooth hemisected and mesial portion used to construct a fixed-fixed bridge thus preventing a free-end saddle prosthetic problem.

Sometimes part of the root canal system is untreatable by either conventional or surgical endodontic means, for example where an instrument has fractured in a root canal and is causing symptoms, or where one of the roots has a traumatic or pathological perfora-tion. Other situations where this operation can be considered occur where the canal cannot be negotiated conventionally and apicectomy with retrograde filling is not possible due to the risk of injury to adjacent structures such as the maxillary sinus or the inferior dental nerve.

162

# 6. REPLANTATION AND TRANSPLANTATION

*Replantation* (or re-implantation) is defined as the replacement of a tooth, after its accidental or deliberate removal from its socket (British Standards Institution, 1969).

The deliberate removal of a tooth that cannot be treated by conventional endodontic techniques, filling its root canal outside the mouth and its immediate reimplantation into its socket is sometimes referred to as *intentional replantation*.

*Transplantation* can be defined as the removal of a tooth (or developing tooth bud) and its replantation into another socket.

Transplantation can be subdivided into *auto-transplantation* (within the same person) or *allo-transplantation* (where the tooth comes from another person).

Transplantation and replantation have been practised for centuries for aesthetic reasons with, generally, unsatisfactory long term results. It is known that the pre-Inca tribes of South America developed great skill in these techniques, and that resection of the apical portion of the root was carried out by them (Weinberger, 1948). Allo-transplantations and replantations were common in the eighteenth century often with fatal results to the recipient because of septicaemia.

Unfortunately, in spite of considerable theoretical, clinical and animal studies, our understanding of the subject is incomplete.


## Replantation

Controversy exists on the best method for the replantation of teeth. Massler (1974) has divided the theories into two groups: those with a cautious and those with a positive approach.

The first group consider that the root of the extracted tooth should be handled very carefully in a swab moistened with sterile saline. The root surface and the attached periodontal fibres and cementum should be preserved and protected from caustic drugs. The tooth should be replanted immediately, and the root canal filled only if the tooth has been out of the mouth for longer than 12 hours. Root tip resection may be necessary so that the tooth seats into its original position. Once in position movement is prevented with a splint such as a periodontal pack. Antibiotics are not considered to be valuable.

The 'positive approach' theorists scrape the root surface to remove debris, 'dead' root fibres and cementum, and also to disinfect the root surface. Replantation is delayed for 3 to 10 days so that the traumatized tissues in the socket have a chance to recover. The tooth is apicected outside the mouth, and a retrograde root filling is placed. It is then replanted until some resistance is felt and is not forcibly pushed into the socket. It is splinted tightly and antibiotics are always prescribed.

On the whole the results obtained by the cautious approach exponents appear to be the more successful and thus an avulsed tooth should be replanted as soon as possible after the accident.

*Technique*

Accidents of this kind are usually reported by telephone and the patient or the parent should be advised to wash the tooth with water and to place it in a wet clean handkerchief. The patient should attend as soon as possible, when the tooth is washed in sterile water and placed in a weak solution of Hibitane. A local analgesic is given and the socket is cleared of blood clot.

The tooth is then washed again and an apicectomy and retrograde root filling performed outside the mouth. Care is taken not to damage the root surface further by holding the tooth by the crown only with a gauze socked in sterile isotonic saline. The tooth is then implanted in the socket gently and slowly to allow fluids to escape from the base of the socket. Care is taken to position the crown correctly, and a check is made to see that it is free of premature contacts with the teeth of the opposing arch.

If the walls of the socket have been expanded during the accident they are now reduced with firm bucco-lingual pressure of the thumb and forefinger.

Splinting of the tooth is essential, and can take the form of interdental wiring and acrylic, or interdental wiring and an acid etch/composite technique if the adjacent teeth are fractured as well and will ultimately require restoration. The splint is removed in 4–6 weeks.

An antitetanus serum injection and an antibiotic cover should be given as soon as possible.

Failure is directly proportional to the time the tooth has been outside the mouth and hence to the degree of desiccation, to the damage sustained by the periodontal ligament, and to the age of the patient—the younger the patient the greater the chances of success. Failure occurs because of progressive and usually rapid external root resorption which becomes evident radiographically some 4–6 weeks after replantation.

Loe and Waerhaug (1961) showed that ankylosis and extensive resorption of roots occurred where the periodontal ligament was removed and minimal resorption with no ankylosis where the periodontal ligament was left intact. Andreasen and Hjørting-Hansen (1966), in a retrospective study, showed that replantation within 30 minutes of avulsion gave the best chances of avoiding resorption.

## Intentional Replantation

This is a useful technique where it is not possible to treat a tooth either by conventional or surgical endodontics and the only other alternative is extraction. Such cases include lower bicuspids with un-negotiable canals and apices in close proximity to the mental foramen.

In such situations the tooth is carefully extracted and without touching the root surface the apex is apicected outside the mouth and a retrograde amalgam filling placed. The socket is irrigated with isotonic saline and the tooth replanted at once. Occlusal adjustment and splinting are carried out as before.

The success of this operation appears to be better than in accidental avulsion and replantation and this is no doubt due to the shorter time that the tooth is outside the mouth and the minimal periodontal injury.

Kingsbury and Wiesenbaugh (1971) reported a 95 per cent success during a 3-year follow-up period and Emmertsen and Andreasen (1966) and Deeb (1968) a 67 per cent success rate after 13 and 2 year follow-up respectively.

## Transplantation

Transplantation is less successful than replantation or intentional replantation and allo-transplantation markedly less successful than auto-transplantations.

At present the subject can be considered experimental and there are very few well documented long term clinical studies available. Hansen and Fibaek (1972) reported on 90 auto- and 54 allo-transplants for up to 15 years. They found that 61 per cent of the auto-transplants and 63 per cent of the allo-transplants were successful after 5 years and this success rate fell to 44 and 33 per cent after 10 years. Root resorption was more prevalent in allo-transplantations. They also noted that root formation continued in teeth with immature roots transplanted autogenically, but did not occur after allo-transplantation.

Because of the uncertain prognosis of all the above techniques interest is now moving towards the use of metal, ceramic and vitreous carbon implants.

## Summary and Conclusions

Whilst replantation and transplantation can be carried out with some degree of success, careful assessment of the situation is essential before submitting the patient to an operation that is usually accompanied by discomfort if not by pain. It may be that the space caused by the loss of one tooth can be better filled with a fixed or removable prosthesis, which will usually be longer lasting and generally less traumatic to the patient.

## 7. ENDODONTIC ENDOSSEOUS STABILIZATION

An endodontic endosseous implant consists of a metallic extension beyond the root apex in order to improve the crown-root ratio and thus stabilize an inadequately supported crown. It has two advantages over the endosseous blade vent, pin or screw implants described by Cherchève (1962), Linkow (1970) and others.

Firstly, once the rubber dam is in position, it is possible to work in a closed system, and instrumentation and insertion of the implant can be carried out in a 'clean' field. Secondly, the implant once sealed in position, has no communication with the oral cavity through the gingival crevice, thus giving the endodontic implant a considerable advantage over other types.

The technique is useful in teeth that have lost bony support in either the coronal or the apical half of the root.

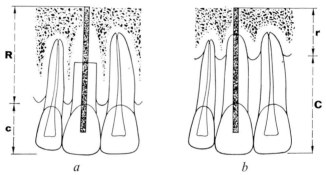

*a*                     *b*

*Fig.* 75. *a*, Where bone loss is in the apical half of the root an endodontic implant improves the root-to-crown ratio (R : c). *b*, Where bone loss is in the coronal half of the root, as in periodontal disease, the root-to-crown ratio remains unfavourable (r : C).

*a. Loss of Bony Support in Coronal Half of Root* (*Fig.* 75*b*)

Bony support loss is usually the direct result of periodontal disease, and if the technique is to be successful it must be reinforced with adequate periodontal treatment. To stabilize a tooth in a diseased periodontium is a waste of time because the disease process will continue with progressive bone loss. In such cases the prognosis of the endodontic endosseous implants is generally poor.

*b. Loss of Bony Support in Apical Half of Tooth* (*Fig.* 75*a*)

The loss of root support may be due to the removal of the apical fragment in a horizontally fractured root which is not amenable to conservative root therapy. It also occurs in teeth with naturally occurring short roots or teeth that have been foreshortened by apical resorption.

It is in these situations that the technique is particularly useful because the gingival crevice is generally healthy, but more importantly because the mechanical advantage and crown root ratio is increased considerably more than it is in the case of bone loss due to periodontal disease (*Fig. 75a*).

The technique was first described in English by Orlay (1960) and refined by Frank (1967). The technique described below is a variation of the Orlay and Frank approach and is an extension of the 'Wiptam' technique described by Harty and Leggett (1972), Leggett (1974). It has three important modifications. Firstly, it is a multi-visit technique, thus allowing the root canal to be débrided and disinfected as well as in conventional root therapy. Secondly, because instrumentation is kept within the canal, in the initial stages, the periapical tissues are not repeatedly disturbed and, thirdly, it is possible to incorporate a core onto the post at the time of implant.

*Technique*

The armamentarium required is similar to that used for the 'Wiptam' post crown technique and consists of Wiptam wire* lengths of 1·3 or 1·5 mm diameter, standardized root canal reamers, engineers' twist drills of 1·30 and 1·50 mm diameter†, two pin vices to hold the twist drills‡, and lengths of 'Wipla' metal tubing§ of which the internal diameter is the same as the Wiptam wire.

Preoperative radiographs, taken at angles 20° mesially and 20° distally to the conventional tube position, are useful in giving an indication of the displacement of the apical fragment relative to the main portion of the tooth.

Local analgesia is usually necessary even if the tooth is non-vital, because the tissue between the fractured portions may be very sensitive.

As in conventional root therapy it is essential that the exact length of the tooth be known and, in this technique, the level at which the fracture occurred. The lengths are calculated by taking a diagnostic wire radiograph with a reamer in position. This reamer is gently introduced into the root canal, through a conventional access cavity, until a resistance is felt. In practice the preoperative radiograph will generally give a good indication of the level to which the diagnostic reamer should be inserted. If the displacement of the two fragments is not great it is possible for the diagnostic reamer to reach to within 1 or 2 mm of the apex of the apical

---

*'Wiptam' clasp wire: Fried. Krupp, Essen, West Germany.
†Dormer Drills 〕Available from any tool shop such as Buck & Ryan,
‡Eclipse Size 122 〕101 Tottenham Court Road, London W1P 0DY.
§'Wipla' tubes: Fried. Krupp, Essen, West Germany.

fragment (*Fig.* 76). If the displacement of the root is such that the root canal is not in line then the diagnostic wire is advanced to a point just short of the fracture.

Provided a radiograph can be taken with an X-ray packet that is not bent in the mouth the length of the tooth and the point at which fracture occurred can be calculated by using the following formula:

$$\text{Length of tooth} = \frac{\text{Length of diagnostic reamer} \times \text{length of tooth on radiograph}}{\text{Length of reamer on radiograph}}$$

The canal should only be instrumented to within 1 mm of the fracture line. It is then enlarged with a twist drill to receive a length of Wiptam wire, which need only fit snugly for 3 or 4 mm short of the fracture.

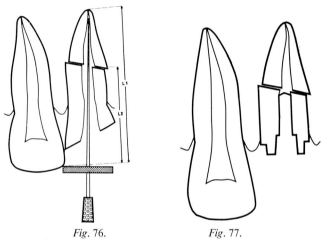

*Fig.* 76.               *Fig.* 77.

*Fig.* 76. Measurement of root canal length where fragment displacement is minimal. From this one can calculate the total length of tooth (L1) and the site of the fracture (L2).

*Fig.* 77. Preparation of root canal just short of fracture line.

The preparation of the post crown is completed and an adequate anti-rotational divide must be cut into the root as this will form the coronal portion of the post (*Fig.* 77).

A length of Wiptam wire is next fitted into the preparation so that it seats in the post hole just short of the fracture line. An impression is taken of the coronal preparation and the protruding wire. The impression technique is immaterial and can be either of the copper ring type or a rubber base impression in a special tray. If the latter technique is used the tray must be so designed that there is sufficient clearance for the rubber impression material to flow and lock around the Wiptam wire (*Fig.* 78).

The post and core implant is constructed in the laboratory in the same manner to a conventional Wiptam post and core. Allowance must, of course, be made for the extension of the post into bone. Thus, the total length of the post should be 2–3 mm longer than the length of both tooth fragments. The calculation of the required post length is made from the diagnostic wire radiograph and the use of the formula given above.

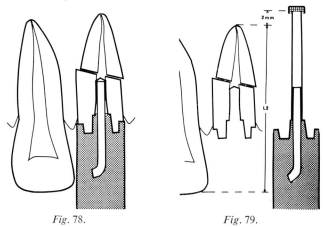

*Fig.* 78.　　　　　　　　　　　　*Fig.* 79.

*Fig.* 78. The impression is similar to that for a post-retained restoration and can be either of compound in a copper ring or in rubber base in a special tray.

*Fig.* 79. Provision for the lengthening of the post in the impression during model construction.

When this measurement is determined a section of Wipla tube is cut to the calculated length above and placed over the Wiptam post in the impression (*Fig.* 79). It is important that the open (and empty) end of the tube is occluded with a small piece of wax in order to prevent plaster from lodging in the tube during the construction of the plaster model. On completion of the model the short Wiptam wire is removed from the tube (which is now incorporated in the model) and replaced with a longer length able to reach the base of the tube.

The anti-rotational device and core are waxed up on the Wiptam wire, which has been grooved to afford mechanical retention, and cast in gold or 'C' metal*. A porcelain jacket is fabricated over the cast core.

The armamentarium required for the surgical operation consists of the normal apicectomy kit to which is added a pin vice and twist drill of the same diameter used in the preparation of the post hole.

---

*'C' metal: Cottrell & Co., Charlotte Street, London W1.

At operation, the fractured apical fragment is exposed and removed. The remaining root requires no preparation except for the removal of any sharp edges. The post hole is lengthened by drilling the remaining dentine between the prepared canal and the fracture line. It is now possible to pass the drill through the root canal until bone is reached at the apex of the socket. Drilling is continued for a further 2 or 3 mm into bone, and this forms a base into which the endosseous implant can be firmly seated. The apical bone cavity is irrigated with normal saline and the implant tried in to make certain that it will seat fully into the prepared bone cavity and also into the coronal preparation. If it does not, either the bony anchorage cavity is deepened or the end of the implant is trimmed with a carborundum disk. When the post and core implant is seen to fit correctly at both its apical and coronal ends it is removed, washed in sterile saline and dried. The apical bony cavity is irrigated and the root canal is dried. A root canal cement is introduced into the deeper portions of the root canal with a reamer and excess cement removed from the coronal area of the preparation. The post is next coated with EBA cement taking care to place cement only on that part of the post that will lie within the prepared canal. This precaution is necessary so that no irritant cement is carried into the bone. The post is placed in the root canal so that it seats correctly in its apical end and also at the root face. The jacket crown may now be cemented onto the core and the post-core-jacket held in position until the cement sets hard. The apical end of the root canal is then inspected and any excess cement removed.

The flap is re-apposed and sutured as in a conventional apicectomy. Splinting is generally not required, but the occlusion must be checked carefully and freed of any contact with the opposing teeth. The patient must also be instructed not to chew in the area for some 2 or 3 weeks. Sutures are removed 4–7 days later (*Fig.* 80).

The weakness of this and other endodontic endosseous implant techniques and indeed of all root canal therapy lies in the inefficiency of the cement seal at the point where the implant protrudes from the root canal. Success in any root therapy depends on the efficiency of the apical seal, and if the seal in the area is inadequate the implant will fail because tissue fluids will find their way into the space between the post and the canal walls where they will stagnate, diffuse into the periapical area and cause an inflammatory reaction.

Amalgam would make an ideal apical seal around the metallic post but it cannot be used because the electrolytic action between the amalgam and the nickel-chrome post will cause corrosion and periapical irritation in the presence of tissue fluids.

In order to overcome the problem of inadequate apical seal various cements have been used. The two most efficient ones appear to be

Ethoxy ortho-benzoic acid (EBA) cement and orthopaedic cement*
which is, in fact, a cold curing acrylic resin. If EBA cement is used
it can serve as both the root filling cement and the luting agent for
the post and core.

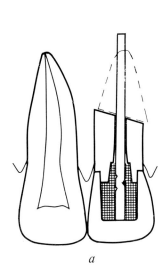
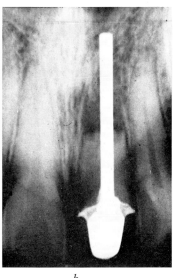

*a*          *b*

*Fig.* 80. *a*, Diagrammatic representation of an endosseous implant.
*b*, Radiograph of an endosseous implant shortly after insertion.

Orthopaedic cement has not been investigated as a cementing
medium in dental implants, but the material is being used in orthopaedic surgery for the cementation of hip prostheses, with considerable success (Charnley, 1970).

REFERENCES

Andreasen J. O. and Hjørting-Hansen E. (1966) Replantation of teeth, I.
Radiographic and clinical study of human teeth replanted after acci-
dental loss. *Acta Odontol. Scand.* **24**, 263.
Andreasen J. O. and Rud J. (1972) Modes of healing histologically after
endodontic surgery in 70 cases. *Int. J. Oral Surg.* **1**, 148.
Blair V. P. and Ivy R. H. (1951) *Essentials of Oral Surgery.* St. Louis,
Mosby.
British Standards Institution (1969) *Glossary of terms relating to dentistry*,
4th ed. British Standard 4492, London.
Charnley J. (1970) *Acrylic Cement in Orthopaedic Surgery.* Edinburgh,
Livingstone.

*C.M.W. Bone Cement: C.W.W. Laboratories Limited, Bone Cement Division,
Clifton Road, Blackpool FY4 4QF.

Cherchève R. (1962) *Les Implants Endo-osseux: technique practique et co-ordonnée d'implantation endo-osseuse en odontostomatologie*. Paris, Maloine.

Deeb E. (1968) Intentional replantation of endodontically treated teeth. In: Grossman L. I. (ed.), *Transactions of the Fourth International Conference on Endodontics*. Philadelphia, University of Pennsylvania, p. 147.

Emmertsen E. and Andreasen J. O. (1966) Replantation of extracted molars: A radiographic and histological study. *Acta Odontol. Scand.* **24**, 327.

Farrar J. N. (1884) Radical and heroic treatment of alveolar abscess by amputation of roots of teeth, with a description and application of the cantilever crown. *Dent. Cosmos* **26**, 135.

Frank A. L. (1967) Endodontic endosseous implants and treatment of the wide open apex. *Dent. Clin. North Am.* p. 675.

Hansen J. and Fibaek B. (1972) Clinical experience of auto and allotransplantation of teeth. *Int. Dent. J.* **22**, 270.

Harnisch H. and Grieger C. (1967) Fehlerquellen bei der Wurzelspitzen-Resektion. *Zahnärztl. Welt* **68**, 125.

Harty F. J. and Leggett L. J. (1972) A post crown technique using a nickel-cobalt-chromium post. *Br. Dent. J.* **132**, 394.

Harty F. J., Parkins B. J. and Wengraf A. M. (1970) The success rate of apicectomy: A retrospective study of 1016 cases. *Br. Dent. J.* **129**, 407.

Hill T. R. (1964) A maxillary labial flap retractor. *Br. Dent. J.* **117**, 172.

Hill T. R. (1967) An amalgam carrier for use in endodontics. *Dent. Pract. Dent. Rec.* **17**, 285.

Hill T. R. (1970) Root canal therapy by means of apicectomy. *Br. J. Oral Surg.* **7**, 168.

Hill T. R. (1974) Surgical endodontics. In: Harty F. J. and Roberts D. H. (eds.), *Restorative Procedures for the Practising Dentist*. Bristol, Wright, p. 204.

Ingle J. I. (1965) *Endodontics*. London, Kimpton, p. 72.

Kingsbury B. C. and Wiesenbaugh J. M. (1971) Intentional replantation of mandibular premolars and molars. *J. Am. Dent. Assoc.* **83**, 1053.

Leggett L. J. (1974) Post crowns. In: Harty F. J. and Roberts D. H. (eds.), *Restorative Procedures for the Practising Dentist*. Bristol, Wright, p. 216.

Leggett L. J. (1975) Personal communication.

Linkow L. I. (1970) Endosseous oral implantology: A 7-year progress report. *Dent. Clin. North Am.* **14**, 185.

Löe H. and Waerhaug J. (1961) Experimental replantation of teeth in dogs and monkeys. *Arch. Oral Biol.* **3**, 176.

Massler M. (1974) Tooth replantation. *Dent. Clin. North Am.* **18**, 445.

Mattila K. and Altonen M. (1968) A clinical and roentgenological study of apicectomized teeth. *Odont. Tidskr.* **76**, 389.

Messing J. J. (1958) Obliteration of the apical third of the root canal with amalgam. *Br. Dent. J.* **104**, 125.

Nordenram A. and Svärdström G. (1970) Results of apicectomy. *Sven. Tandläk. Tidskr.* **63**, 593.

Orlay H. G. (1960) Endodontic splinting treatment in periodontal disease. *Br. Dent. J.* **108**, 118.

Roberts D. H. and Sowray J. H. (1970) *Local Analgesia in Dentistry*. Bristol, Wright, p. 52.

Rothschild M. B. (1970) The use of bone wax to facilitate retrograde filling techniques. *J. Br. Endodont. Soc.* **4**, 60

Rud J. and Andreasen J. O. (1972) Operative procedures in periapical surgery with contemporaneous root filling. *Int. J. Oral Surg.* **1**, 297.

Rud J., Andreasen J. O. and Möller-Jensen J. E. (1972) *Endodontic Surgery: A Histologic, Radiographic and Clinical Study*. Reprinted from: *Int. J. Oral Surg.* **1**, 148, 161, 195, 215, 258, 272, 297, 311. Copenhagen, Munksgaard.

Selden H. S. (1970) Bone wax as an effective hemostat in periapical surgery. *Oral Surg.* **29**, 262.

Stallard R. E. (1973) Periodontic-endodontic relationships. In: Siskin, M (ed.), *The Biology of the Human Dental Pulp*. St. Louis, Mosby, p. 376.

Tschamer H. (1955) Cas Ergebnis der Nachkontrolle von 160 Wurzelspitzenamputationen. *Zahnärztl. Rdsch.* **64**, 432.

Weinberger B. W. (1948) *An Introduction to the History of Dentistry*. St. Louis, Mosby.

Wengraf A. (1964) Radiologically occult bone cavities. *Br. Dent. J.* **117**, 532.

# CHAPTER 9

# ENDODONTICS IN CHILDREN

ENDODONTICS in children has to be considered separately from adult root therapy because the anatomy and pulp physiology of the primary and developing permanent dentition differs from the mature dentition. The aims are, of course, identical, i.e. to retain the permanent teeth in function indefinitely and the primary dentition until it is shed normally.

As was seen in Chapter 3 the deciduous teeth have proportionally much larger pulps and thinner enamel and dentine than the permanent teeth (*Fig.* 30). There is no clear demarcation between the pulp chamber and root canal and the pulp horns are more pointed. Multi-rooted deciduous teeth show a greater number of inter-connecting branches and Winter (1962) has found that radiographs reveal an abundance of lateral canals in the inter-radicular area. Both deciduous and permanent immature teeth have wide open and funnel-shaped apical foramina, so that the pulp receives a rich and abundant blood supply with consequent improved healing if injured.

Physiologically, the deciduous pulp has a formative function and, during tooth development, dentine is deposited at a fairly rapid rate. The role of the pulp in the mature deciduous tooth changes and now assumes a resorptive function.

For these reasons, the approach to children's endodontics must be different from that to the fully mature dentition.

The subject will be discussed under the following headings:

1. Pulp capping of vital deciduous pulps.
2. Partial pulpectomy of vital deciduous teeth
   i. With calcium hydroxide
   ii. With 'tissue fixing' (mummifying) pastes.
3. Root therapy of non-vital deciduous teeth.
4. Treatment of immature permanent teeth:
   i. Vital teeth with open apices (partial pulpectomy)
   ii. Non-vital teeth with open apices.
5. Surgical treatment.

## 1. PULP CAPPING OF VITAL DECIDUOUS PULPS

Pulp capping, as defined by the *Glossary of Terms relating to Dentistry* (British Standards Institution, 1969) consists of the application of one or more layers of protective materials over an exposed vital

174

pulp. The subject is controversial and some authorities dispute its value. To have any chance of success the exposure to be capped must be small, clean, and the pulp must not be contaminated. This limits the technique to accidental traumatic exposures in teeth with very little caries.

In such cases the exposed pulp is quickly covered with an inert or mildly antiseptic material such as calcium hydroxide or zinc hydroxide and eugenol, and the 'pulp cap' is protected with a layer of stiff quick-setting zinc oxide, the final restoration being placed over this lining at the same visit.

Technically the procedure is difficult because it is seldom possible to keep the site of exposure free from saliva contamination. Further, the pulp chambers of deciduous teeth are large in relation to crown size and often there is not enough space to place a pulp cap, a lining and an adequate permanent restoration.

Hobson (1970a) considers that the response of the deciduous pulp to caries is similar to that which occurs in permanent teeth, but the involvement of the coronal pulp alone occurs infrequently, both coronal and radicular pulps being generally diseased. Unlike the mature permanent pulp the deciduous pulp undergoes irreversible pathological changes long before its exposure. She also suggests that if adverse signs and symptoms have occurred, including exposure, the pulp is markedly inflamed and when an irreversible change had occurred in the coronal portion of the pulp it will probably have occurred in the radicular pulp as well.

For these reasons, once exposure or any other signs and symptoms have occurred, there is little chance of preserving the vitality of the whole pulp by capping or the radicular pulp by pulpotomy.

## 2. PARTIAL PULPECTOMY (VITAL PULPOTOMY) OF VITAL DECIDUOUS TEETH

A partial pulpectomy is the removal of the coronal portion of a vital pulp endangered by disease, with the object of maintaining the health of the remaining (radicular) portion of the pulp. The operation is also commonly referred to as 'pulpotomy' or 'vital amputation' and both these terms are deprecated (British Standards Institution, 1699).

Partial pulpectomy is considered the treatment of choice in deciduous teeth with exposed vital pulps and also in immature permanent teeth.

There are two techniques associated with this operation. In the first, calcium hydroxide is used in the hope that the amputated radicular pulp will remain vital, and in the second, the amputated portion is 'fixed' with a medicament such as formocresol.

175

### a. *Partial Pulpectomy with Calcium Hydroxide (Fig.* 81)

When the local analgesic, which is essential for this technique, is seen to be effective, the tooth is isolated, preferably with a rubber dam, and the caries excavated. The roof of the pulp chamber is carefully removed with a sterile excavator or a slowly rotating medium size round bur. The contents of the pulp chamber are removed with a sharp sterile excavator so that the orifices or the root canals

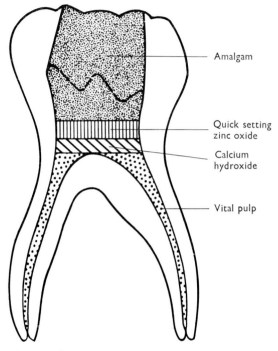

Amalgam

Quick setting zinc oxide

Calcium hydroxide

Vital pulp

*Fig.* 81. Partial pulpectomy (vital pulpotomy) with calcium hydroxide.

are visible. The resultant haemorrhage is arrested by irrigation with sterile saline, distilled water or analgesic solution and gentle blotting with sterile cottonwool pledgets. Haemorrhage is generally not a problem and ceases after about two minutes. Calcium hydroxide is then applied to the amputated pulp either as a freshly mixed paste of calcium hydroxide powder and sterile saline or in one of the proprietary pastes of calcium hydroxide in methyl cellulose (Pulpdent, Calxyl, Reogan). The pulp cap is protected by flowing a creamy layer of quick setting zinc oxide over the calcium hydroxide, taking care not to force it into the radicular pulp. A permanent amalgam restoration is inserted at once to protect the pulp from salivary contamination. The success rate of the technique is difficult to determine, for some researchers report a low success rate (Via, 1955; Law, 1956) whilst others report a relatively high success (Sawyer and Amaral, 1954; Cooke and Rowbotham, 1956; Jeppesen (1971).

Via (1955), Hannah and Rowe (1971) and Rule (1974) consider that failure in many cases can be attributed to internal resorption, which is most frequently found near the junction of the coronal and radicular pulp. For this reason, the technique below is generally favoured and has had a higher success rate than that using calcium hydroxide alone.

### b. Partial Pulpectomy with
### 'Tissue Fixing' (Mummifying) Medicaments (Fig. 82)

Several medicaments have been suggested and of these formocresol and pastes containing a proportion of paraformaldehyde are in common use. *Formocresol\**, which is a solution of 19 per cent formaldehyde and 35 per cent cresol in a glycerin/water vehicle, was introduced by Buckley in 1905 and described by Sweet in 1930. The technique was reintroduced as a two visit procedure, by his son (Sweet, 1963). Redig (1968) modified the technique so that only one visit was required and both techniques have a very high success rate.

As before, the coronal pulp is amputated at pulp chamber floor level and the haemorrhage arrested. In the one visit technique, the solution is carried to the tooth on a pledget of cottonwool and left in contact with the pulp for five minutes. In the two visit technique, a lightly dampened pledget of cottonwool is sealed into the pulp chamber for about seven days.

In both techniques the cottonwool is then replaced with a layer of zinc oxide mixed with equal parts of eugenol and formocresol. This layer is covered with a lining of quick setting zinc oxide and the tooth restored, at once, with a permanent restoration.

Medicaments containing paraformaldehyde are also useful in partial pulpectomy cases. Hobson (1970b) formulated a devitalizing and mummifying paste† containing—

| | |
|---|---|
| Paraformaldehyde | 1·00 g |
| Lignocaine | 0·06 g |
| Propylene glycol | 0·50 ml |
| Carbowax 1500 | 1·30 g |
| Carmine | 10·00 mg |

*Buckley's Formocresol: Crosby Laboratories, 3010 West Burbank Blvd, Burbank, California 915105, U.S.A.
†Boots Pure Drug Co. Ltd., Nottingham, U.K. Dispensed under Code E.13498.

The pulp chamber is prepared as before and a small layer of paste (about 1 mm³) carried to the exposed tissue on a pledget of cotton-wool. This is sealed in by flowing, over the cottonwool, a layer of quick setting zinc oxide cement of creamy consistency. After seven days, the protecting temporary filling and devitalizing paste is removed and the pulp cavity is partially filled either with Putridemors 22* (containing thymol, cresol and iodoform in a zinc oxide base) or a lining of zinc oxide mixed with equal parts of eugenol and formo-cresol. The tooth is permanently restored with amalgam.

ONE-VISIT TECHNIQUE

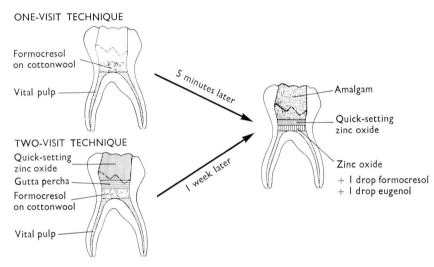

Formocresol on cottonwool

Vital pulp

5 minutes later

TWO-VISIT TECHNIQUE

Quick-setting zinc oxide

Gutta percha

Formocresol on cottonwool

Vital pulp

I week later

Amalgam

Quick-setting zinc oxide

Zinc oxide
+ I drop formocresol
+ I drop eugenol

*Fig.* 82. Partial pulpectomy (vital pulpotomy) with 'tissue fixing' medicaments.

Hannah and Rowe (1971) reported a 5-year study of vital pul-potomies carried out using the following materials: N2, calcium hydroxide, zinc oxide/eugenol alone or in combination with paraffin or paraformaldehyde and paraffin. Of the 151 teeth treated with the N2 method 98 per cent were successful. They did point out, however, that histological studies showed that the pulp, after satis-factory initial fixation and devitalization, is resorbed and replaced by ingrowing granulation tissue, which eventually becomes inflamed on reaching the hardened dressing, and this suggests that the method is not suitable for permanent teeth.

Comparison of techniques using the other materials showed that pulpectomies with paraformaldehyde containing medicaments gave superior results to zinc oxide/eugenol or calcium hydroxide.

*Putridemors 22: Via B. Cellini 16, Milan 20129, Italy.

### c. *Devitalizing Technique* (*Fig.* 83)

The above two techniques assume that effective local analgesia can be obtained so that the coronal portion of the pulp can be removed. However, this is not always possible, either because the child will not accept local analgesia or because the analgesic may not have worked satisfactorily. In such instances, a two visit technique can be employed. As a first stage the coronal portion of the pulp is devitalized and this is followed, some 10–14 days later, with a

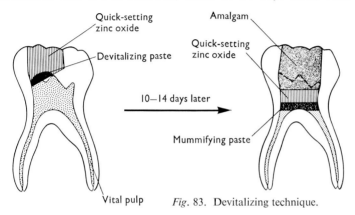

Quick-setting zinc oxide

Devitalizing paste

Amalgam

Quick-setting zinc oxide

10–14 days later

Mummifying paste

Vital pulp

*Fig.* 83. Devitalizing technique.

procedure that mummifies the pulp remnants. At the initial appointment, the carious cavity is gently excavated so that the exposed pulp is visible. If the excavation is carried out carefully the procedure can be entirely pain-free. The devitalizing paste, on a pledget of cottonwool, is placed on the exposure. This operation is delicate as the paste must be placed on the exposure with sufficient pressure to bring it into contact with the exposed pulp and yet gentle enough to prevent the paste from being pushed forcefully into the radicular pulp with painful consequences.

The cottonwool and paste are then covered with a creamy mix of quick setting zinc oxide which is flowed on so that no pressure is exerted on the pulp. When the first protective layer has set, the cavity is filled with a temporary dressing. Care must be taken that the devitalizing paste is hermetically sealed from the gingival tissues because, if it leaks, tissue destruction may result.

The choice of devitalizing paste is wide but it is preferable to use a paste containing lignocaine because this reduces the slight pain sometimes experienced for one or two days. Examples of commonly used devitalizing pastes are the Hobson paste mentioned before and 'Toxavit'.*

---

*Toxavit: Lege Artis Manufacturing Co., D-7 Stuttgart 1, PO Box 992, West Germany.

Devitalizing pastes containing arsenic should *never* be used, for arsenic is a protoplasmic poison which can cause massive tissue destruction if it inadvertently comes into contact with gingival tissue through leakage of the temporary filling.

At the second visit, some 10–14 days later, an aseptic pulpal necrosis should have occurred. The cavity is re-excavated, the pulp chamber cleared of necrotic debris, irrigated and, without instrumenting the root canals, a mummifying agent is placed over the root canal orifices to control any residual infection. A lining is placed over the mummifying paste and the tooth restored, either with amalgam or, if badly carious, with a stainless-steel crown.

The choice of mummifying paste is wide and most contain paraformaldehyde and sometimes tricresol as well. Examples of two such pastes are the Kri-I paste* and Gysi's trio paste†.

### 3. ROOT THERAPY OF NON-VITAL DECIDUOUS TEETH (*Fig.* 84)

Sometimes this operation is referred to as 'non-vital pulpectomy' or 'pulpotomy'. Strictly speaking these terms are incorrect for both imply the removal of part or all of the vital dental pulp.

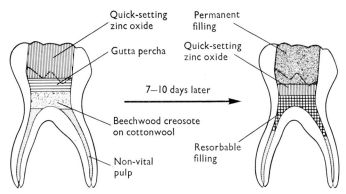

*Fig.* 84. Root canal therapy of non-vital deciduous tooth.

The treatment of such teeth is usually a two visit procedure. On the first visit the carious cavity and the pulp chamber are cleared of all caries and necrotic tissue. The root canals are cleaned, as well as possible, with barbed broaches. The pulp cavity is irrigated, preferably but not necessarily with an antiseptic solution such as chloramine 'T', and disinfected with beechwood creosote which is

---

*Kri-I Paste: Pharmachemie A.G., 8053 Zurich, Switzerland.
†Gysi's Trio Paste: Amalgamated Dental Distributors, 26–40 Broadwick Street, London W1A 2AD.

carried to the pulp chamber on a pledget of cottonwool, damped (not soaked) in the medicament. It is important that no excess liquid be allowed to remain in the chamber because it is moderately toxic and irritant to tissue. Since it is a mixture of creosol, guaicol and other phenols, beechwood creosote has one important advantage in that it is mildly analgesic as well as antiseptic.

The dressing is sealed in the pulp chamber for 7–10 days when it is replaced with a filling of zinc oxide mixed with equal parts of eugenol and formocresol, or alternatively, with a resorbable iodoform paste such as Kri-I. This filling is covered with a quick setting zinc oxide and the tooth is restored permanently either with amalgam or with a stainless-steel crown. The technique is applicable to most non-vital deciduous teeth. However, if undrained pus is present apically, then it may be wise if the carious cavity and pulp chamber were cleared of caries and necrotic debris and the abscess allowed to drain for 48 hours. The excavated pulp chamber should be protected against food impaction with a light cottonwool dressing. Generally, it is neither necessary nor desirable (because of food impaction) to allow the tooth to remain open for longer than 48 hours and treatment, as outlined above, can start if there are no other adverse symptoms.

## 4. TREATMENT OF IMMATURE PERMANENT TEETH

One of the most difficult problems in endodontic therapy is the treatment of permanent teeth with incompletely formed apices, and until about 20 years ago treatment was unsatisfactory, and usually led to tooth loss. The object of the treatment, as in conventional root therapy, was the hermetic sealing of the apical foramen, and two alternatives were available. In the first, the apex was approached through a conventional coronal access cavity, which was wasteful of tooth substance because of the large root canal diameter. The canal was instrumented with files and could very seldom be prepared satisfactorily in the apical third because of the appreciable divergence of the canal walls. Another problem was the eggshell thinness of the root in the apical third which made instrumentation difficult and perforation likely (*Fig.* 85). Gutta percha points were then rolled between glass slabs in order to obtain a point of sufficient thickness to occlude the apex. Because of the canal divergence, it was seldom possible to obtain an adequate apical seal. The operation was very time consuming and usually not appreciated by the young patient.

The second technique was essentially a 'through-and-through' root filling (*see* p. 156) after exposing the root apex surgically. Apart from the trauma of surgery on a young child, the operation was not entirely satisfactory because the thinness of the root apically necessitated resection to a level where the amalgam or other root filling could be packed against 'solid root'. This foreshortened an already short root to such a degree that satisfactory post retained restoration became almost impossible.

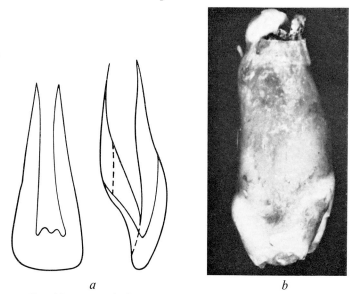

*a*             *b*

*Fig.* 85. *a*, Developing permanent upper central incisor. Note divergence of root canal apically and the eggshell thinness of root in in this area. *b*, Failed root therapy in developing incisor. Note perforation of root buccally and the failure of the calcific barrier across the open apex because of over-filling. (*Courtesy of Dr. J. W. Cunningham*).

Current treatment aims at promoting normal root growth or, at least, apical repair with calcific tissue and is often successful in both vital and non-vital teeth.

### *a. Vital Teeth and 'Open Apices' (Fig.* 86)

Treatment is essentially a partial pulpectomy as already described on p. 175. The pulp is amputated at the cervical level which normally coincides with the constriction of the canal at a point where the coronal and radicular pulp segments meet. The degree of haemorrhage is often a good indication of pulpal health. Bleeding should cease in two or three minutes if the severed pulp is not traumatized further and only gently blotted with the blunt ends of sterile paper points or cottonwool. If bleeding is minimal it is likely that the pulp is already degenerating, and if bleeding is excessive and continues for five or six minutes it is safe to assume that the pulp is

182

inflamed with considerable vasodilatation. In either event it may be wise to remove a further portion of pulp, thus bringing the amputated portion closer to the apex where it is likely that the morphology and function will be near normal (Stewart, 1962). When the bleeding is arrested, the pulp is covered with a layer of calcium hydroxide, as described on p. 176.

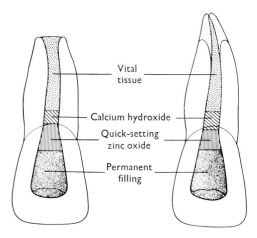

*Fig.* 86. Root canal treatment of vital tooth with open apex.

Normally, a dentine bridge can be seen about 6–8 weeks postoperatively and the apex continues to form normally.

An annual clinical and radiographic check must be kept on teeth treated in this manner, not only to check on the normal development of the root apex but also the check for pulp necrosis or a progressive calcification of the root canal which may occur in a small number of cases. This calcification begins in the coronal area of the pulp and extends apically. Calcification, once it has begun, normally proceeds rapidly and may block the major portion of the canal. If this happens subsequent conventional root therapy and post crown preparation become very difficult. For these reasons conventional root therapy should be instituted as soon as calcification of the root canal begins.

### b. *Non-vital Teeth with Open Apices (Fig.* 87)

In theory it is not possible for root apex formation to continue unless the epithelial root sheath of Hertwig retains its specialized function. Thus reports of continued 'normal' root formation in teeth deemed to be non-vital are suspect. However, as Dylewski (1971)

183

has shown, it is possible for the apical area to be invaded by connective tissue which becomes calcified and continuous with the predentin at the apex. The mechanism is not clearly understood and further studies are required.

It is also possible that a tooth that has been classified as non-vital on the evidence of pulp vitality testing alone may, in fact, contain some vital tissue apically, and this can often be demonstrated by instrumentation. In these cases, it is possible that the apex continues to form if the vital tissue is not destroyed by over-zealous instrumentation or by toxic medicaments. Several authors have reported successful root formation in non-vital teeth of children (Cooke and Rowbotham, 1960; Ball, 1964; Rule and Winter, 1966; Steiner et al., 1968; Dylewski, 1971).

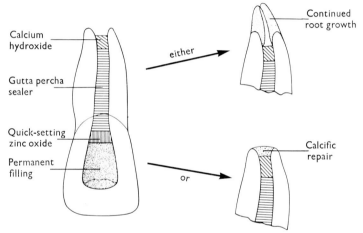

*Fig.* 87. Root canal treatment of non-vital tooth with open apex.

Van Hassel and Natkin (1970) report apical closure of a premolar in a 37-year-old patient.

In all these reports the root filling technique is generally the same, although there is conflicting opinion about the medicaments used to irrigate, dress and obturate the canal.

The root canal is cleared of necrotic tissue by irrigation and the walls prepared usually with files alone because of its wide lumen. Accurate early root canal length determination is essential so that the instrumentation is confined to the root canal and kept just short of the apex. This is necessary so that any apical vital or granulation tissue is not disturbed. Irrigation should be with saline or sterile water only so that the specialized apical tissue is not damaged (Rule and Winter, 1966). The canal is then dried and dressed, either with an antibiotic paste or with a mixture of calcium hydroxide and camphorated parachlorophenol. Of these, the former is preferred because it is relatively bland and is less likely to cause tissue damage. The canal is sealed with a pledget of cottonwool and a quick setting zinc oxide cement.

The tooth is not filled permanently until it is symptomless and several dressings may be necessary. On the final appointment the canal is irrigated with saline and dried with blunt-ended paper points. The apex is sealed with a paste of calcium hydroxide or a mixture of calcium hydroxide and camphorated parachlorophenol. The deposition of the paste at the correct level and in contact with the apical tissues is not an easy procedure. Slowly rotating lentulo spiral fillers are commonly used but careful control is necessary if the paste is not to be forced past the apical foramen. Celluloid 'Jiffy' tubes* are sometimes advocated, but again, placement and control of the paste is difficult.

A more effective method of introducing paste sealers into the root canal is by the use of specially designed endodontic syringes with a screw plunger. The paste is deposited, through a relatively wide bore needle, by the rotation of the screw plunger. Hypo-Cal† is an example of a calcium hydroxide preparation available in such a syringe made of plastic.

A sturdier and more useful syringe was developed by Greenberg & Katz and described by Krakow and Berk (1965). This consists of a barrel screw type plunger, two wrenches and an assortment of needles ranging in size from gauge 13 to 30. The advantage of this instrument is that it can be used with various sizes of needle, thus allowing its use even in fine canals. Also, since 400 pounds pressure per square inch can be developed within the instrument, it is now possible to introduce really thick mixes of calcium hydroxide or sealer into the root canals. The paste need only occlude 2–3 mm of canal, the remainder being filled with gutta percha and sealer, which can be removed easily should a post crown be required at a later date.

Valuable experimental work on the developing incisors of primates is being carried out by Torneck and Smith (1970) and Torneck et al. (1973a, b and c). Their results show that removal of most of the pulp and immediate sealing of the access cavity led to a retarded and irregular root formation. When there was a partial pulp removal there was an accelerated rate of foraminal closure by irregular dentine without a proportionate increase in root length. They also demonstrated that continued root growth and foraminal closure was often seen despite the presence of pronounced inflammatory changes in both the residual pulp and the periapical tissue.

---

*Odus Dental A.G., Dietikon, Zurich, Switzerland.
†'Hypo-Cal': Ellman Dental Mfg. Co. Int., PO Box 68, Cedarhurst, N.Y. 11516.

The efficacy of camphorated parachlorophenol alone or as a paste when mixed with calcium hydroxide was investigated, and it was found that the use of parachlorophenol alone was detrimental to apical formation and suggested that this is so because of the high irritating potential of the material.

On the other hand, the use of calcium hydroxide/camphorated parachlorophenol used as a thick paste appeared to accelerate the rate at which apical growth and foraminal clossure occurred.

In the above study the efficacy of calcium hydroxide alone has not been tested, but Massler (1972) concludes that calcium hydroxide is the material of choice in direct pulp-capping techniques, and this is the view held by Winter and Rule (1974) who advise the use of a calcium hydroxide paste in the apical filling of non-vital teeth with incomplete apices.

The radiographic appearance of apical repair is seen as an increase in length or, in cases where the epithelial sheath of Hertwig is destroyed, as an irregular calcific barrier across the open apex (*Fig.* 87). In either case, when repair is complete, the canal should be reinstrumented and a well condensed root filling should be inserted.

## 5. SURGICAL TREATMENT

If, in spite of all the above conservative treatment, root end closure does not occur, then the only alternative is surgical interference with either a 'through-and-through' or a retrograde root filling (*see* Chapter 8). As already mentioned, apicectomy further reduces the available length of an immature tooth and makes post crown restoration more difficult.

REFERENCES

Ball J. S. (1964) Apical root formation in a non-vital immature permanent incisor: Report of a case. *Br. Dent. J.* **116**, 166.
British Standards Institution (1969) BS 4492. *Glossary of Terms relating to Dentistry*, 4th ed. London.
Cooke C. and Rowbotham T. C. (1956) A review of a technique for pulpotomy and report on 175 cases. *Br. Dent. J.* **100**, 174.
Cooke C. and Rowbotham T. C. (1960) Root canal therapy in non-vital teeth with open apices. *Br. Dent. J.* **108**, 147.
Dylewski J. J. (1971) Apical closure of non-vital teeth. *Oral Surg.* **32**, 82.
Hannah D. R. and Rowe A. H. R. (1971) Vital pulpotomy of deciduous molars using N2 and other materials. *Br. Dent. J.* **130**, 99.
Hobson P. (1970a) Pulp treatment of deciduous teeth. I, Factors affecting diagnosis and treatment. *Br. Dent. J.* **128**, 232.
Hobson P. (1970b) Pulp treatment of deciduous teeth. II, Clinical investigation. *Br. Dent. J.* **128**, 275.

Jeppesen K. (1971) Direct pulp capping on primary teeth: A long-term investigation. *J. Int. Ass. Dent. Child.* **2**, 10.

Krakow A. A. and Berk H. (1965) Efficient endodontic procedures with the use of the pressure syringe. *Dent. Clin. North Am.* p. 387.

Law D. B. (1956) An evaluation of vital pulpotomy technique. *J. Dent. Child.* **23**, 40.

Massler M. (1972) Therapy conducive to healing of the human pulp. *Oral Surg.* **34**, 122.

Redig D. F. (1968) A comparison and evaluation of two formocresol pulpotomy technics using 'Buckley's' formocresol. *J. Dent. Child.* **35**, 22.

Rule D. C. (1974) Special consideration in children's dentistry. In: Harty F. J. and Roberts D. H. (ed.), *Restorative Procedures for the Practising Dentist.* Bristol, Wright, p. 372.

Rule D. C. and Winter G. B. (1966) Root growth and apical repair subsequent to pulpal necrosis in children. *Br. Dent. J.* **120**, 586.

Sawyer H. F. and Amaral W. J. (1954) Use of calcium hydroxide as a pulp capping material: A clinical study in young adults. *U.S. Armed Forces Med. J.* **5**, 1155.

Steiner J. C., Dow P. R. and Cathey G. M. (1968) Inducing root end closure of non vital permanent teeth. *J. Dent. Child.* **35**, 47.

Stewart D. J. (1962) Delayed pulpotomy in traumatised teeth. *Br. Dent. J.* **113**, 305.

Sweet C. A. (1930) A procedure for treatment of exposed and pulpless deciduous teeth. *J. Am. Dent. Assoc.* **17**, 1150.

Sweet C. A. (1963) Formocresol technique. In: Grossman L. I. (ed.), *Transactions of the Third International Conference on Endodontics.* Philadelphia, University of Pennsylvania, p. 32.

Torneck C. D. and Smith J. S. (1970) Biologic effects of endodontic procedures on developing incisor teeth. I, Effect of partial and total pulp removal. *Oral Surg.* **30**, 258.

Torneck C. D., Smith J. S. and Grindall P. (1973a), Biologic effects of endodontic procedures on developing incisor teeth. II, Effect of pulp injury and oral contamination. *Oral Surg.* **35**, 378.

Torneck C. D., Smith J. S. and Grindall P. (1973b) Biologic effects of endodontic procedures on developing incisor teeth. III, Effect of debridement and disinfection procedures in the treatment of experimentally induced pulp and periapical disease. *Oral Surg.* **35**, 532.

Torneck C. D., Smith J. S. and Grindall P. (1973c) Biologic effects of endodontic procedures on developing incisor teeth. IV, Effect of debridement procedures and calcium hydroxide-camphorated parachlorophenol paste in the treatment of experimentally induced pulp and periapical disease. *Oral Surg.* **35**, 541.

Van Hassel H. J. and Natkin E. (1970) Induction of foraminal closure. *J. Dent. Assoc. S. Afr.* **25**, 305.

Via W. F. (1955) Evaluation of deciduous molars treated by pulpotomy and calcium hydroxide. *J. Am. Dent. Assoc.* **50**, 34.

Winter G. B. (1962) Abscess Formation in connexion with deciduous molar teeth. *Arch. Oral Biol.* **7**, 373.

Winter G. B. and Rule D. C. (1974) Personal communication.

CHAPTER 10

# PERIODONTAL DISEASE AND THE DENTAL PULP

by J. Saville Zamet, M.Phil., F.D.S. R.C.S.

*Senior Lecturer, Department of Periodontology, The Royal Dental Hospital, London*

THE fact that poor oral hygiene, with accumulation of dental plaque, is the cause of both dental caries and periodontal disease is well established. Less well accepted is the association between periodontal and pulpal disease. Both are common and many teeth are affected by both. Inflammation and degeneration or necrosis was found in the pulps of 90 per cent of teeth with periodontal disease and restorations (Bender and Seltzer, 1972). Instances of failure in treating periodontal pockets and in endodontic therapy may be due to inadequate diagnosis of the dual involvement—one tissue being treated and the other ignored.

## PULPAL PERIODONTAL COMMUNICATIONS

The possibility that periodontal disease might be related to or cause pulpal disease was reported by Colyer (1924) and Cahn (1927), who described structures which are termed lateral canals. Cahn stated: 'It does not require a wide stretch of the imagination to see how easily an infective process might spread from without inwards, rapidly involving the pulp, especially in teeth having these side canals.' By means of indian ink perfusion studies Kramer (1960) and Cohen et al. (1960) demonstrated a vascular communication via these channels. They represent an original communication between the developing dental sac and the dental papilla, with the majority being present in the apical half of the root, except in the case of multi-rooted teeth where numerous communications exist in the area of furcation (Seltzer and Bender, 1965). Histologic studies also revealed that lateral canals may become sealed by the formation of cementum and that these 'sealed' canals may be inadvertently opened by instrumentation during periodontal therapy, with exposure of the pulp. The vessels running in lateral canals do not provide a major source of collateral circulation, although they contribute to the overall nutrition of the pulp. However, they do provide a major communication between the pulp and the periodontal ligament and vice versa (Langeland et al., 1974). Disease in either may rapidly spread from one to the other. It is of critical

188

importance to be sure whether the initial lesion is of endodontic or periodontal origin. The classification of these lesions suggested by Simon et al. (1972) will be used as the basis for discussion.

1. *Primary Endodontic Lesions* (*Fig.* 88*a*)

Clinically these lesions may appear concurrently with drainage from the gingival sulcus and/or swelling in the buccal attached gingiva. The impression is that these lesions are of periodontal origin. In reality they are sinus tracts resulting from a necrotic pulp draining coronally through the periodontal ligament. Inflammation from a

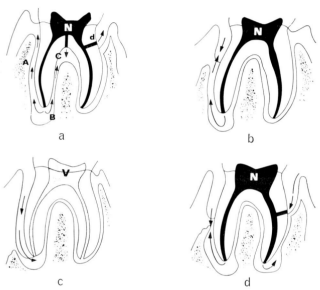

a  b  c  d

*Fig.* 88. *a*, Primary endodontic lesions: (A) pathways extending from apex via periodontal ligament space to gingival sulcus, apex to bifurcation (B), lateral canal to bifurcation (C) and lateral canal to periodontal pocket (d). *b*, Primary endodontic lesion with secondary periodontal involvement. *c*, Primary periodontal lesion extending to apex. *d*, Primary periodontal lesion with secondary endodontic involvement. via a lateral canal (right side of tooth). Combined perio-endo lesion joined by two separate lesions coalescing (left side). N, Non-vital pulp. V, Vital pulp.

necrotic pulp may alternatively extend from the apex of the tooth into the bifurcation area, mimicking the appearance of periodontal involvement. Direct extension of inflammation from the pulp may occur into the bifurcation when lateral canals are present. When an accessory canal is present some distance from the apex on the mesial or distal surfaces of a tooth, extension of disease from the pulp into the attachment tissues may give the clinical and radiographic appearance in an infrabony pocket.

189

2. *Primary Endodontic Lesions with Secondary Periodontal Involvement (Fig. 88b)*

If treatment is delayed to the primary endodontic lesion it may become secondarily involved with periodontal breakdown. Inflammatory periodontal disease occurs primarily in the gingival unit, the major cause being bacterial plaque.

It often spreads into the area of crestal bone with accompanying apical proliferation of the epithelial attachment from enamel onto the cemental surface of the tooth. With the development of periodontitis detachment of the proliferating epithelium from the root surface occurs with the formation of pockets. Active crestal bone loss is also apparent on radiographic examination. The tooth now requires both endodontic and periodontal therapy.

3. *Primary Periodontal Lesions (Fig. 88c)*

These lesions are caused by periodontal disease. The process of chronic periodontitis gradually progresses along the root surface until the apical region is reached. The presence of occlusal trauma resulting from parafunctional habits may on occasions join with local inflammation as a co-destructive factor (Glickman, 1965). Under these circumstances inflammation extends along altered pathways into the periodontal ligament, with the formation of vertical infrabony defects.

4. *Primary Periodontal Lesions with Secondary Endodontic Involvement (Fig. 88d)*

As periodontal lesions progress towards the apex, lateral or accessory canals may be exposed to the oral environment, which leads to necrosis of the pulp. Pulpal necrosis may also result from periodontal procedures where the blood supply through an accessory canal, or the apex, is severed by the action of a curette.

5. *Combined Lesions (Fig. 88d)*

Combined lesions occur where an endodontic lesion progressing coronally becomes continuous with a periodontal lesion progressing apically. The ultimate picture is indistinguishable from the other two lesions mentioned previously.

## PERIO/ENDO SYNDROME

This can be defined as a syndrome involving inflammation or degeneration of the pulp, with a clinical pocket on the same tooth. Such a syndrome can be initiated by either pulpal or periodontal disease (Bender and Seltzer, 1972). The predisposition is for molar teeth, but less so in single rooted teeth, since the distribution of lateral canals occurs more frequently in molars.

## Differential Diagnosis

1. PAIN: Periodontal disease is not usually accompanied by pain. The exceptions, such as periodontal abscess or necrotizing ulcerative gingivitis, only produce pain of a moderate degree. The symptoms of severe pain are most likely to be of endodontic origin.

2. SWELLING: In teeth with pulpal involvement the swelling is seen apical to the mucogingival junction in alveolar mucosa. In periodontal abscess formation the swelling tends to be within the zone of attached gingiva or close to the gingival margin on the palatal mucosa. Swelling on the face may occur in teeth with endodontic involvement, but is rarely observed in teeth with periodontal disease.

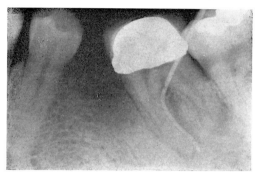

*Fig.* 89. Primary endodontic lesion: A gutta percha point in situ demonstrating the pathway of infection from the apex of the mesial root of the lower left second molar into the bifurcation.

3. SINUS TRACTS: Where a sinus tract opens into the gingival sulcus the origin of the lesion can be determined by the insertion of either a gutta percha point or diagnostic wire (*Fig.* 89). The gutta percha point has the advantage that being pliable it can follow a tortuous pocket around the root of the tooth. Sinus tracts of endodontic origin are often narrow, accepting only one wire or gutta percha point, periodontal lesions are often more broad based (Bender and Seltzer, 1972).

## Radiographic Examination

Periodontal lesions with endodontic involvement and endodontic lesions with periodontal involvement and combined lesions may be impossible to differentiate on the radiograph, but differences sometimes occur.

A necrotic pulp may cause a sinus tract to extend from the apex coronally through the periodontal ligament along the mesial or distal tooth surfaces. This lesion appears as a greyish radiolucency extending along the entire root length. If the crestal bone level, mesially and distally, appears to be normal and only the bifurcation area is radiolucent, then the suspicion must be one of pulpal involvement. Similarly, an area of radiolucency in relation to one isolated furcation, with all other areas being normal, would again point to endodontic exploration being carried out first. Endodontic lesions in relation to healthy teeth or teeth with shallow restorations should point towards the presence of periodontal disease, or occlusal trauma. Compulsive bruxism may result in necrosis of the pulp, especially in relation to mandibular incisor teeth (Ingle, 1960).

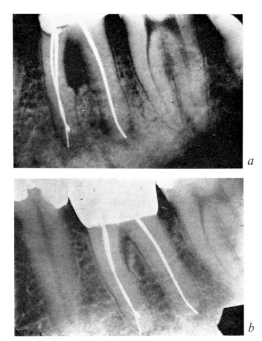

*a*

*b*

*Fig.* 90. Primary endodontic lesion: *a*, Appearance of a molar tooth immediately following root canal therapy. A necrotic pulp draining into the bifurcation had resulted in considerable bone loss. *b*, The same tooth two years later showing complete filling-in of the defect.

## TREATMENT

*Primary Endodontic Lesions*

These lesions usually heal following root canal therapy. The sinus tract into the gingival sulcus disappears at an early stage once the necrotic pulp has been treated (*Fig.* 90). If the lesion has not healed within six months and there is no reduction in the size of the apical radiolucency, then periodontal surgery should be instituted.

192

*Primary Endodontic Lesions with Secondary Periodontal Involvement (Fig. 91).*

The prognosis for the tooth will depend on the success of the periodontal therapy, on the assumption that the endodontic procedures are more certain of success.

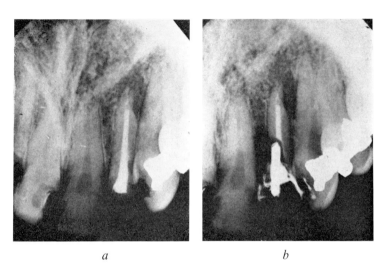

*a*          *b*

*Fig.* 91. Primary endodontic lesion with secondary periodontal involvement. *a,* Root-filled lateral incisor prior to restoration. The supporting tissues are healthy. *b,* Post crown preparation with perforation of the root mesially. Secondary periodontal breakdown has occurred with loss of crestal bone.

The endodontist to all intents and purposes is dealing with a six-walled or sometimes five-walled intrabody pocket. He is also working in a 'closed' system, once the rubber dam is in place, and a complete regeneration of apical bone will usually occur. Periodontal therapy has none of these advantages, the system being 'open' with continual bacterial reinfection through the gingival sulcus or pocket. Alveolar bone loss is, in most cases, permanent, although further destruction can be prevented.

*Primary Periodontal Lesions (Fig. 92), Primary Periodontal Lesions with Secondary Endodontic Involvement (Fig. 93) and Combined Lesions*

ANTERIOR TEETH: In single rooted teeth the prognosis is often poor because of the degree of periodontal breakdown the exception being where the periodontal defect is formed by a three-walled intrabony pocket. The diagnosis of a three-walled intrabony pocket, however, cannot be made clinically or radiographically and if the

193

possibility exists an exploratory surgical procedure will be required. Root canal therapy, however, must be completed before periodontal intervention.

Following the completion of root canal therapy, the area is anaesthetized and reverse bevel flap incisions are made both labially and palatally, starting at the gingival margin and ending at the alveolar crest. Full thickness mucoperiosteal flaps are raised. All chronic inflammatory tissue is curetted away in the defect down

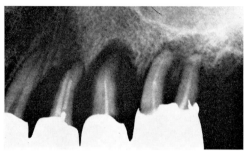

*Fig.* 92. Primary periodontal lesions. Chronic periodontitis has progressed to the root apices on premolar and molar teeth.

to bone. The exposed root surface is planned to remove the surface layer of cementum. Fenestrations are made through the sclerosed wall of the defect into the surrounding cancellous bone using a half-round bur. The predictability of 'bone fill', especially where the lesion is broad based, can be increased by the use of an autogenous cancellous bone graft, tuberosity, retromolar or extraction sites providing donor material. The flaps are then replaced and accurately sutured interdentally. The surgical area is covered with periodontal dressing for one week. The sutures are then removed. The use of antibiotics over a 5-day period is recommended in these cases.

POSTERIOR TEETH: Where an individual root is hopelessly involved with loss of alveolar support, amputation may be considered, removing the involved root at the point where it joins the crown. The other alternative is to hemisect the tooth mesiodistally or buccolingually in maxillary molars and from buccal to lingual in mandibular molars, the involved root or roots being removed.

### Indications for Root Removal

#### 1. *Advanced Periodontal Disease*

The pattern of alveolar and supporting bone loss in periodontal disease may be unequal, even in relation to the different roots of a molar tooth. If left untreated, the adjacent healthier root support would become involved by direct extension of the periodontal lesion.

194

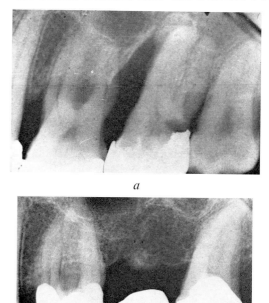

*a*

*b*

*Fig.* 93. Primary periodontal lesion with secondary endodontic involvement: *a*, Chronic periodontitis extending to the apices of mesial and palatal roots of a non-vital maxillary second molar. A carious lesion is also present distally. *b*, The severe degree of bone loss, impossibility of instrumenting into the exposed but narrow furcation and the close proximity of the disto-buccal root of this tooth to the third molar combine to give a negative prognosis. It was therefore extracted and a fixed bridge was constructed.

An attempt at correction by osseous surgery would also lead to the loss of supporting bone around adjacent roots. Removal of the offending root will allow the tooth to be retained and for a return of a normal clinical and radiographic appearance. Pocket depths that are well beyond the mucogingival junction may not allow for predictable treatment with a re-establishment of a functional zone of attached gingiva. Sacrifice of such a root may simplify the surgical approach.

## 2. *Close Root Proximity*

Roots of teeth that are in tight proximal position that do not permit access for oral hygiene, do not allow for normal gingival form. This type of situation is often found where the distobuccal root of the

195

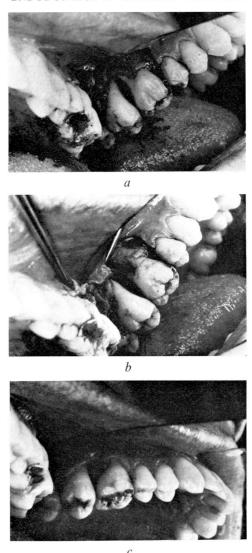

*a*

*b*

*c*

*Fig.* 94. *a,* A vertical bony defect extending between the converging roots of the maxillary first and second molar teeth. *b,* the disto-buccal root of the first molar has been amputated and the area curetted free of granulation tissue and transseptal fibres. When bone loss in this area is severe, the mesio-buccal root of the second molar may be treated in a similar fashion. The defect will 'fill' like a socket. *c,* The area of root amputation is carefully streamlined into the adjoining crown and root surfaces. Ancillary methods of plaque control are helpful in these areas, i.e. the proxa brush (Butler), the interspace brush or, in difficult areas, pipe cleaners.

196

first maxillary molar flares towards the mesiobuccal root of the second maxillary molar (*Figs.* 94, 95). In addition to the problems of plaque removal, no space remains for an adequate embrasure area if the teeth are to be restored. Selective root removal will allow for the re-establishment of a proper embrasure area.

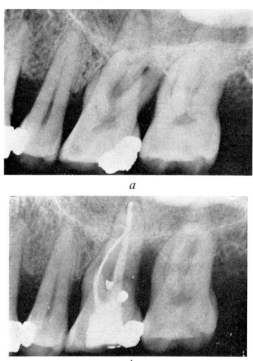

*a*

*b*

Fig. 95. *a*, Vertical alveolar bony defect related to closely approximated roots between maxillary first and second molars. The furcation was probeable buccally and distally, but not mesially. *b*, Root canal therapy was carried out on the mesio-buccal and palatal roots of the first molar. The disto-buccal root was amputated and the opening into the pulp chamber sealed with amalgam.

3. *Furcation Involvement*

As a sequel to periodontal disease, the furcation of molar teeth may become exposed. The small defect that can be probed is often misleading, a much larger space being formed by the housing of the furcation between the roots. Such areas are not amenable to plaque control and are often the site of periodontal abscess formation. Root removal allows access to these areas and careful preparation and restoration of the remaining portion of the tooth will allow for adequate plaque control.

197

## Contra-indications for Root Removal

1. Where plaque control following the initial preparation phase of periodontal treatment still remains poor.

2. Decreased bony support in relation to all roots of the involved tooth, with an unfavourable crown-to-root ratio.

3. Fused roots.

4. Short thin roots.

5. A furcation area placed apically to the extent that considerable supporting bone would have to be sacrificed to expose it.

6. Surrounding anatomy that would preclude the formation of a functional band of attached gingiva round the remaining roots.

7. When root removal would result in inadequate support for a tooth that was acting as a terminal abutment for a fixed prosthesis.

8. Endodontically inoperable canals in remaining roots, where retrograde amalgam restorations are impossible.

9. Where adequate restorations cannot be carried out on teeth where root removal is proposed.

## Root Amputation

Whenever possible, endodontic therapy should be carried out first prior to root removal. Coronal reshaping and buccal-lingual narrowing should also be done first to bring occlusal pressure over the solid roots that remain. If thought advisable the involved teeth may be splinted to adjacent teeth.

The need for root removal may become apparent during diagnosis and treatment planning of the case, as a solution to treating roots with extensive periodontal breakdown. Endodontic treatment is completed on the tooth in question as soon as the patient's plaque control has reached a satisfactory level and the inflammatory phase has been resolved. Full thickness mucoperiosteal flaps are reflected to expose the furcation area. In relation to maxillary molars, this needs careful exploration with a probe to be sure that the furcation is not exposed on all three surfaces. If so, the prognosis is extremely poor. The cut in the root is made with a 701 L (I.S.O. No. 012 L) bur, which is long enough to reach from one side of the root to the other. Care is taken to maintain correct angulation of the bur, so as not to damage the remaining root(s) or the crown. Removal of some of the buccal cortical plate of bone may be required so that the separated root can be gently elevated out of its socket, care being taken not to apply pressure to the adjacent tooth or bone.

Once the root has been removed, the area of the stump should be reshaped with diamond stones, so that it blends imperceptibly into the remaining tooth structure. Enough clearance should also be left between the undersurface of the crown and the gingival tissue to allow for adequate plaque control. The tooth surface should be finally finished with fine diamond stones and then polished.

A re-evaluation of the periodontal situation is carried out some three months following root removal. If mucogingival and osseous deformities are present in this quadrant of the mouth, definitive periodontal surgery is now carried out.

An alternative method of treatment allows for resection to be carried out at the time of periodontal surgery. This has the advantage of allowing for only one surgical procedure on the area. The disadvantage is that bony healing has yet to occur and the extent to which this will progress cannot always be predicted and this may result in more radical reshaping in the area than might otherwise be required.

The necessity for root removal may not be found until flaps are reflected for the purpose of periodontal surgery. In this situation the root may be separated and removed, despite the fact that endodontic treatment has not been carried out. A cavity is cut over the pulp stump with an inverted cone bur and a dressing of calcium hydroxide placed over the exposed pulp. Definitive endodontics can be carried out at a later stage, after the periodontal dressings have been removed.

*Hemisection (Fig. 96)*

In this technique the resection is carried through the crown of the tooth and the involved root, with its part of the crown, is removed. Hemisection is the technique to be preferred where teeth are to be included in a fixed prosthesis (Abrams and Trachtenberg, 1974). A considerable advantage is achieved if the initial crown preparation is completed first. This then serves as a guide to entering the furcation. Endodontic treatment is always carried out prior to root removal.

The tooth is sectioned with a 702 L (I.S.O. No. 016 L) bur. In maxillary molars one root may be removed by either buccopalatal or mesiodistal sectioning, the other two roots being retained providing the furcation is not open. If the furcation proves to be open mesially, buccally and distally all three roots should be separated and the one with the best support retained (Hamp et al., 1975). Mandibular molars are sectioned buccolingually into two halves. In teeth where the furcation is open, the bur can be introduced into the furcation and separation is simple. Where the furcation is not exposed and filled with bone, full thickness mucoperiosteal flaps should be reflected buccally and lingually to gain access. It is also important to make the cut at the expense of that portion which is to be removed. This minimizes the risk of over-cutting the retained section.

Confirmation that the section has completely gone through the tooth may be obtained by gently trying to wedge the segments apart to see if movement occurs. If doubt still exists a radiograph may provide confirmation. When the section is complete the involved part of the tooth is extracted with forceps. In finishing the preparation it is important to remove the overhang of the crown at the

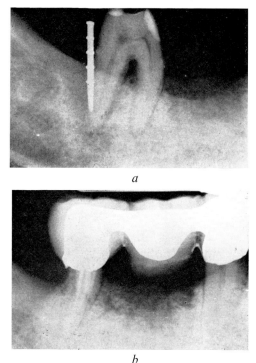

*a*

*b*

*Fig.* 96. *a*, A vertical bony defect on the distal of the mandibular second molar with a Hirschfeld silver point in situ. The bifurcation is also involved. *b*, Root canal therapy has been carried out on the mesial root. The tooth was then hemisected and the mesial root used as an abutment for a fixed bridge.

bifurcation and to blend the cut surface of the stump into the retained portion of the tooth. The remaining part of the tooth is restored with a full crown, either as an individual tooth or as part of a fixed prosthesis.

Healing following root removal may leave a gingival contour that is far from ideal. This may either take the form of a deep dimple or rolls of gingival tissue in the embrasure area, where a root has been amputated. These areas are readily reshaped by gingivoplasty to allow for good plaque control.

200

BIBLIOGRAPHY

Abrams L. and Trachtenberg D. I. (1974) Hemisection—technique and restoration. *Dent. Clin. North Am.* **18**, 415.

Bender I. B. and Seltzer S. (1972) The effect of periodontal disease on the pulp. *Oral Surg.* **33**, 458.

Cahn L. R. (1927) The pathology of pulps found in pyorrhoetic teeth. *Dent. Items Int.* **49**, 598.

Cohen D. W., Keller G., Feder M. and Livingston E. (1960) Effects of excessive occlusal forces in gingival blood supply. *J. Dent. Res.* **39**, 677.

Colyer F. (1924) Bacteriological infection in pulps of pyorrhoetic teeth. *Br. Dent. J.* **45**, 558.

Glickman I. (1965) Clinical significance of trauma from occlusion. *J. Am. Dent. Assoc.* **70**, 607.

Hamp S. E., Nyman S. and Linder J. (1975) Periodontal treatment in multi rooted teeth. *J. Clin. Periodontol.* **2**, 126.

Ingle J. I. (1960) Alveolar osteoporosis and pulpal death associated with compulsive bruxism. *Oral Surg.* **13**, 1371.

Kramer I. H. R. (1960) The vascular architecture of the human dental pulp. *Arch. Oral Biol.* **2**, 177.

Langeland K., Rodrigues H. and Dowden W. (1974) Periodontal disease bacteria and pulpal histopathology. *Oral Surg.* **37**, 257.

Seltzer S. and Bender I. B. (1965) *The Dental Pulp.* Philadelphia, Lippincott.

Simon J. H. S., Glick D. H. and Frank A. L. (1972) The relationship of endodontic/periodontic lesions. *J. Periodontol.* **43**, 202.

Stallard R. E. (1972) Periodontic/endodontic relationships. *J. Oral Surg.* **34**, 314.

# CHAPTER 11

# PROBLEMS IN ENDODONTIC TREATMENT

## I. EMERGENCY TREATMENT

IT is axiomatic that a patient in pain must be rendered comfortable as soon as possible. The practice of treating the patient with antibiotics and analgesics without attempting to discover and remove the cause of the pain is bad practice.

In the endodontic field, patients present as an emergency due to one of three conditions, i.e.:

1. Acute pulpitis
2. Acute periodontitis
3. Acute apical abscess.

In each case the emergency treatment consists of applying one or more of the basic surgical principles, and these are:

1. Remove the cause of pain
2. Provide drainage if fluid exudate is present
3. Rest the affected part
4. Prescribe analgesics if appropriate.

### 1. *Acute Pulpitis*

The causes of pulp injury, its prevention and treatment have been discussed in Chapter 4. The question is often asked, At what stage should palliative treatment cease and be replaced by pulp extirpation? Ideally the treatment should be related to the histopathological state of the pulp but it is impossible to determine this without exposing the pulp. The clinician thus relies on the history given by the patient and on the visible signs.

As a rule of thumb, if a tooth becomes painful without an exciting factor such as hot, cold, sweet food or trauma or wakes the patient at night then it is likely that the pulp has been irreversibly injured and pulp extirpation is indicated.

It may be difficult to anaesthetize an acutely inflamed pulp and this has been discussed on p. 204.

### 2. *Acute Apical Periodontitis*

This can be defined as an acute inflammation of the periodontal ligament. It is often a direct result of irritation through the root canal or from trauma to the tooth, and generally, but not always, associated with an acute pulpitis.

As exudate is not present periapically the treatment consists of removing any pulp remnants, irrigating, drying the canal and sealing in a sedative and disinfecting dressing. Care must be taken not to injure the periapical tissues further by probing past the apex or by medicating the canal with an irritant drug which may diffuse periapically and compound the injury.

Corticosteroid preparations, such as 'Ledermix' paste (triamcinolone acetonide) or *Septomixine** have also been found to be very effective in relieving the acute phase. Both these medications are placed in the canal short of the apical foramen, and presumably diffuse into the periapical tissues to control the inflammatory process.

The tooth will probably be slightly extruded and the occlusion must be relieved by grinding the opposing tooth or teeth. The importance of this stage in the treatment of the patient can not be over-emphasized and the occlusion should be checked routinely whenever the patient is seen.

### 3. *Acute Apical Abscess*

This condition develops as a sequel to an apical periodontitis and the differential diagnosis of the two states may be difficult. Radiography is not helpful as the lesion does not become radiographically visible until one or both cortical plates become eroded. A positive diagnosis cannot be made until the canal contents are investigated.

Where a swelling exists the diagnosis and treatment are generally easier. Relief can be obtained speedily by relieving the occlusion and obtaining drainage. The practice of prescribing an antibiotic without obtaining drainage is incorrect and prolongs the patient's misery unnecessarily.

Opening into the pulp chamber may cause considerable pain because of vibration. This can be minimized by stabilizing the tooth with the fingers and obtaining access by using a very small round bur in a turbine. The pulp chamber should be cleared, as far as possible, of necrotic tissue and debris by instrumentation and irrigation. If the tooth is exceedingly periostitic and/or there is a copious discharge of exudate then it should be left on open drainage for at least 48 hours. At the end of this period the patient should be seen again and, if comfortable, the access cavity enlarged and the canal instrumented, irrigated and cleaned conventionally.

It is important that the root canal be cleaned, medicated and sealed as soon as possible so that food does not pack into the canal and cause an acute flare up. The practice of leaving the canal open for weeks, if not months, has nothing to commend it and usually

---

*Septomixine-Specialités Septodont, 29 Rue des Petites-Ecuries, Paris (10ᵉ), France.

leads to periodic 'flare-ups' due to food blocking the access cavity, and often to caries of the pulp chamber and root canal, and this makes the root therapy and subsequent restoration of the tooth very difficult.

If a tooth so treated is symptomless whilst on open drainage but flares up as soon as it is sealed then one must question the thoroughness of the débridement. This is probably the commonest cause of postoperative flare up for no tooth will 'settle' unless the canal is thoroughly cleaned. It is also possible that a tooth adjacent to that being treated is non-vital and has a periapical area of infection in communication with the first tooth. Drainage of this second area occurs through the root canal of the first tooth. However, as the root canal of the second tooth has not been cleaned it continues to be a source of infection and this causes the 'flare up' as soon as the discharge path is blocked. As a precaution two teeth on either side of any obviously non-vital tooth should be routinely tested for vitality prior to any endodontic treatment.

Periapical tissues may also be irritated by caustic medicaments particularly if carried to the canal on a paper point whose tip is allowed to pass through the apical foramen. Paper points are useful for drying canals and for carrying medicaments into them but there is no advantage in sealing them in root canals.

Sometimes because of anatomical difficulties or because there is an immovable obstruction to the root canal it may not be possible to obtain drainage through the canal. In such instances the treatment will depend on the presence or absence of swelling and both these situations have been discussed on pp. 141–144.

## II. INADEQUATE ANALGESIA DURING PULP EXTIRPATION

Profound analgesia is essential for vital pulp extirpation, yet there are occasions where, in spite of the correct dosage and technique, the analgesia obtained is inadequate. Such occasions are traumatic to the patient and embarrassing to the dentist.

The reasons for failure are numerous and whilst the topic is of great importance in endodontic therapy it cannot be considered in detail in a Handbook of this size. The subject has been considered fully in Roberts and Sowray's *Local Analgesia in Dentistry* (1970) under the following headings: *a*. Failure of analgesia in a tooth with an acutely inflamed pulp; *b*. Failure of infiltration analgesia; *c*. Failure of regional analgesia.

The reasons for failure are enumerated below and the reader is referred to the above-mentioned book for a fuller discussion of each topic.

### 1. *Failure of Analgesia in a Tooth with an Acutely Inflamed Pulp*

Such a tooth is generally periostitic and it may be impossible to achieve analgesia of sufficient depth. The reason for this failure is unknown although various theories have been propounded. These include the following:

  *a.* The pain due to the periostitic tooth produces so many nerve stimuli that the local analgesic solution is unable to block the conduction of all these impulses and some of them manage to reach the brain.

  *b.* The pH of the inflammatory products in the region of the tooth is more acidic than usual, thus making the local analgesic solution less effective.

  *c.* Jorgensen (1960) has postulated that as there is a tendency for pain to neutralize in the central nervous system the effects of analgesics such as morphine, there may be a similar explanation for the poor results achieved with local analgesics.

  *d.* Hudson (1960) has mentioned the theory of a possible spread of inflammation along the myelin sheaths of the nerve which restricts the absorption of the local analgesic.

  *e.* There is usually increased vascularity of the tissues surrounding the periostitic tooth and hence the local analgesic is removed by the bloodstream before it is able to work. Nearer the apex there is vascular stasis so that the analgesic is unable to reach it.

### 2. *Failure of Infiltration Analgesia*

This may be due to one or a combination of the following:

*a. Deposition of Analgesic Solution in the Wrong Area during a Supraperiosteal Injection*

The analgesic solution should always be placed supraperiosteally and as nearly over the apex of the tooth as possible. This can be assessed from the position of the crown. A common error is to infiltrate too far away from bone or too deeply into soft tissue when the solution is liable to pass intramuscularly which, apart from causing failure of analgesia, will also result in after-pain.

*b. Wrong Assessment of the Dosage required*

The amount of analgesic solution must be assessed correctly, the dosage required depending on the thickness and density of the bone through which it has to pass. This varies with—

  i. *The patient:* If he is well built and has a heavy bone structure then a larger dosage will be required than if he is small and frail. Males tend to need more analgesic than females.

ii. *Local anatomy:* A larger dose is required where the root lies comparatively deeply in relatively dense bone. For example, the maxillary canine will require more analgesic than the upper second molar whose root is more superficial and lies in bone that is less dense than that surrounding the canine.

*c. Incorrect Choice of Technique*

Analgesia which may be fully adequate for an extraction may be of insufficient depth for routine conservation, and pulp extirpation demands more profound analgesia than either conservation or extraction. Apicectomy also requires a deep level of analgesia, possibly because of the infection usually present around the apex of the tooth. Where deep prolonged analgesia is required, regional analgesia will often prove more satisfactory than an infiltration technique.

*d. Incorrect Technique in the Presence of Inflammation or Infection*

An analgesic is usually ineffective in the presence of inflamed tissue, the reason for this being unknown. It is thought that the altered pH of inflamed tissues may inactivate the solution, but another factor could be the increased irritability of the nerve fibres. Where inflammation is present an infiltration injection should be avoided and either a regional nerve-block used or a general anaesthetic administered.

*e. Intravascular Injection*

Although this complication may occur during any infiltration injection, it is particularly likely to happen when injecting in the upper second or third molar regions or when giving an inferior dental block. If this occurs one may see a sudden pallor of the face and often the patient will either feel faint or lose consciousness. Although an aspirating syringe should be used to prevent intravascular injection, if one inserts the needle and injects very slowly then the blood vessels usually contract before the needle reaches them, thus avoiding this complication. As soon as the patient shows any sign that an intravascular injection is being given, the needle should be partially withdrawn to remove it from the lumen of the blood vessel before administering any further analgesic solution.

*f. Variation in Individual Tolerance to the Analgesic Solution*

Individuals vary considerably in their degree of resistance to the achievement and duration of local analgesia. Thus one may have a particular patient who never requires more than 0·5 ml for any infiltration injection, whereas another may invariably require at least 2 ml. Similarly, the duration of analgesia may vary between individuals from 20 minutes to 6 hours with the same amount of analgesic. Therefore it is desirable to note on the patient's record card the type, quantity, and strength of analgesic used. This is particularly important when the patient varies considerably from the norm.

*g. Variation in the Pain Threshold of Individuals and even the Same Individual on Different Occasions*

The degree of pain tolerance varies very widely with different individuals, and the sensation which one may interpret as pain another would merely consider discomfort. Obviously in the former a far deeper level of analgesia is required. To lower the pain threshold premedication is sometimes indicated and this may be administered intravenously (*see* Chapter 2). The tolerance of any one individual varies quite considerably from time to time due to such factors as systemic disease, domestic worries, tiredness or hunger.

### 3. *Failure of Regional Analgesia*

Most of the factors responsible for an infiltration injection failing to achieve analgesia also apply to a regional nerve block. However, the most important factor is the deposition of the solution in the wrong site which may be due to several causes:

*a.* Insufficient knowledge of the local anatomy of the region.

*b.* Individual anatomical variations occurring in different patients, especially those factors affecting the relative position of the mandibular foramen.

*c.* Variations due to age: for example, in children the mandibular foramen is relatively lower than in adults.

*d.* Faulty technique. With the inferior dental nerve-block the commonest errors are—

  i. Injecting too far posteriorly because the barrel of the syringe is not far enough back over the opposite premolars.

  ii. Injecting too low down. This is often because the lower lip is allowed to lie between the barrel of the syringe and the teeth, thus giving it a downward angulation.

### *Alternative Techniques*

In practice, failure to obtain analgesia is an infrequent occurrence and when it does occur it is likely to be in the mandibular posterior teeth. One must accept that an acutely inflamed pulp will remain exquisitely painful in spite of what appears to be a satisfactory inferior dental nerve block.

In such infrequent instances several alternative techniques are available and these are:

i. Sedation of the pulp and postponement of instrumentation.

ii. Intra-osseous injection.

iii. Pressure analgesia.

iv. Mummification techniques.

v. General anaesthesia.

*a. Sedation of the Pulp and Postponement of Instrumentation*

The kindest treatment to the patient is to accept the failure of the local analgesia, dress the pulp to reduce the inflammation and attempt analgesia on a subsequent occasion.

The pulp may be sedated with eugenol or with mixtures of essential or artificial oils. One such commercially available preparation is: 'Chlorbutanol'*.

The hyperaemic pulp bleeds copiously on exposure and it should be allowed to do so for some two to three minutes as it reduces intrapulpal pressure. The exposure is then covered with a loose pledget of cottonwool soaked in one of the medicaments mentioned above. The cottonwool is covered with a soft mix of quick setting zinc oxide which is flowed onto the cottonwool so that there is no pressure on the exposed pulp. Ideally the zinc oxide should be covered with a permanent filling so that inadvertent chewing on the tooth will not force the dressing into the pulp chamber with painful consequences for the patient.

The corticosteroid-antibiotic preparations have been discussed on p. 51 and these are useful alternative dressings in teeth with inflamed pulps. The application of a corticosteroid such as 'Ledermix'†, in paste form, affords almost instantaneous relief by reducing pulp inflammation. It is generally assumed that the corticosteroid acts by constricting the enlarged blood vessels of the inflamed pulp and that if the medicament is left in contact with the pulp for longer than 72 hours the pulp will become non-vital due to blood stasis. In the author's experience this does not happen and in certain instances the pulp has remained vital some six months after the application of Ledermix paste. Therefore on the subsequent visit an analgesic should again be given and when it is effective the pulp extirpated as in the case of the pulp sedated with eugenol or other essential oils.

---

*Produit Dentaires S.A., Vevey, Switzerland.

†Lederle Laboratories, Cyanamid of G.B. Ltd., Bush House, London WC2.

208

*b. The Intra-osseous Injection*

In this technique a hole is drilled in cortical bone so that an analgesic solution can be deposited into the cancellous bone from where it will rapidly diffuse to the apices of one or two teeth, thus affording profound but short-acting analgesia.

The technique is described fully in Roberts and Sowray (1970) and consists of drilling a hole through the cortical plate of bone with a spiral twist drill, a Beutelrock or a specially designed van den Bergh drill. A needle, whose diameter is very slightly less than the needle used to drill the hole, is then used to deposit the analgesic solution in the cancellous bone between the roots of adjacent teeth. The near perfect fit of the needle in the previously drilled hole prevents 'backflow' of solution. If drill and needle are not matched then it is necessary to use a rubber seal around the needle or a long hub with a short needle so that an effective seal is formed around the needle and 'backflow' of solution prevented.

This technique leads to instantaneous analgesia without soft tissue involvement and has a very high success rate. However, it has disadvantages in that it is more complex to perform, is of very short duration and, most importantly, there is a risk of introducing infection into the cancellous bone, either by imperfectly sterilized instruments or by injecting through infected tissues. Further, if periapical infection is present (for example, where a multi-rooted tooth has one or more canals vital and the remainder gangrenous) there is a danger that this infection will be forced to a different site within the bone by the pressure with which the analgesic solution is injected.

*c. Pressure Analgesia*

In this technique analgesia is obtained by using pressure to force an analgesic (either cocaine crystals or a paste of crystalline procaine powder) into the exposed vital pulp.

Caries is carefully removed from the cavity and the paste or crystals placed over the exposure. A piece of gutta percha, large enough to fill the cavity, is warmed and placed over the analgesic. A large amalgam plugger is then used to compress the gutta percha and thus propel the paste or crystals into the pulp. The patient experiences momentary pain and, in theory, pulp analgesia should be immediate and profound.

The technique has disadvantages in that the resulting analgesia may be partial and a second or third attempt may be necessary before the entire pulp can be extirpated. Secondly, and of greater importance, there is a risk of forcing infected material, either from the pulp chamber or from a gangrenous canal, into the periapical tissues. This latter possibility is unacceptable and places the technique in a dubious category.

Another pressure analgesia technique consists of injecting the pulp with a local analgesic solution. In this technique the needle is advanced into the pulp chamber and a few drops of solution injected. This technique is painful and not very effective because the back flow of solution is considerable. Sometimes it is suggested that gutta percha be packed into the cavity in order to prevent back flow and thus increase the injection pressure.

As before there is a risk of forcing infected material into the periapical tissues and the criticisms made above apply to this technique as well.

### d. Mummification Techniques

Devitalization and mummification techniques have been discussed in Chapter 9 in relation to endodontics in children. These same techniques can be used on a pulp where analgesia is inadequate after repeated attempts or where it is inadvisable to use an injection technique. For example, in haemophiliacs or in patients who are allergic to any one of the drugs in analgesic solutions.

The pulp is devitalized as described on p. 179. As in the deciduous dentition one application of devitalizing paste may not be sufficient to devitalize the entire pulp. In such instances a second application of devitalizing paste may be required. This is necessary because, in the adult dentition, the entire pulp cavity has to be instrumented, and, ultimately, filled with a non-resorbable root filling. It will be recalled that this is not necessary in deciduous teeth for, by choice, the root filling is of the resorbable variety and vital deciduous pulp remnants are left in situ and mummified.

Choice of devitalizing pastes has been discussed on p. 179 and, again, it must be emphasized that pastes containing arsenic should never be used because of the tissue destruction that can occur if arsenic comes in contact with the peridental tissues.

### e. General Anaesthesia

There are rare and exceptional cases where a general anaesthetic is the only way a vital pulp can be extirpated. Generally the reasons are not related to the failure of local analgesia but rather to the attitude of the patient. In such instances, before embarking on such a course, the operator must satisfy himself that the tooth is of sufficient importance to the patient's well-being and that the patient will accept subsequent endodontic and restorative procedures without recourse to further general anaesthetics which place the patient at risk (McEwan, 1974).

There are, of course, occasions when a general anaesthetic is essential to obtain drainage of a non-vital tooth that is so painful that any manipulation of the tissues is otherwise impossible.

## III. RADIOGRAPHY

Radiography is an invaluable aid to endodontic therapy and without it the quality of treatment would be very much poorer. However, radiographs can be misleading particularly if examined in a cursory manner so that essential diagnostic features are overlooked (*Fig.* 97).

It must be remembered that the radiograph gives limited information because it is the shadow of the object under investigation and for shadows to become discernible there must be adequate contrast between them. This may be difficult to achieve. Further, a radiograph is a two dimensional picture of a three dimensional object, and superimposition and loss of detail is to be expected.

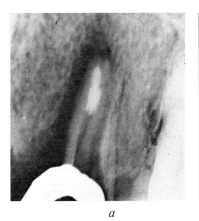 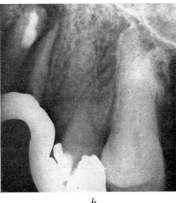

*a*          *b*

*Fig.* 97. *a*, Radiograph showing an apparently satisfactory sectional root filling. *b*, Radiograph taken from a different angle showing vertical fracture line.

Before considering what can be seen on a radiograph it is as well to recall what can *not* be seen. A pulp with acute pulpitis looks identical, on the radiograph, to a normal healthy pulp. Similarly there is no difference in the X-ray appearance of a vital and a necrotic pulp within the tooth, but the latter will ultimately cause periapical changes which are visible on the X-ray. These take the form of an initial thickening of the periodontal ligament which may ultimately develop into a visible periapical radiolucent area.

Sometimes there may be visible changes within the pulp cavity in a tooth whose pulp is chronically inflamed. These changes are evidence of pulp calcification and thus visible on the X-ray as pulp stones or a generalized 'gravelling'. Alternatively such a pulp may produce root resorption which is easily seen on the radiograph.

It is well known that a tooth with an acute abscess will show no periapical bone changes on the radiograph for some weeks after the initial symptoms. Bender and Seltzer (1961), Regan and Mitchell (1963) and Wengraf (1964) have shown experimentally that the removal of cancellous bone is not detectable on X-ray and that the lesion does not become radiographically visible until one or both cortical plates becomes involved.

Thus an acute periapical abscess will not show on a radiograph and it is normally assumed that any periapical exudate or pus fills the narrow spaces between the trabeculae which remain unaltered. Wengraf (1964) points out that whilst this may be true it is an unnecessary assumption for even were the medullary spaces totally eroded the lesion would still remain radiologically occult.

Often one looks for a continuous lamina dura on the X-ray as evidence of pulp health. If this can be seen then it can safely be assumed that the pulp is vital because the roots of teeth generally lie within the cortical plates and any alteration to the lamina dura is generally visible on X-ray. However, the corollary is not true, i.e. if an X-ray picture shows a deficient lamina dura it does not necessarily follow that peridental disease is present. As Manson (1963) has pointed out the lamina dura, seen as a white line on the radiograph, represents the plate of bone which lines the tooth socket and this bone will only show on the X-ray if the rays pass through it tangentially. Thus if the angulation of the X-ray is not favourable the lamina dura may not be visible on the X-ray. Generally it is safer to look for the shadow of the peridontal ligament because this is not affected, to the same degree, by the angulation of the X-ray beam. A healthy peridontium is seen on the radiograph as a continuous uniform black line between the root surface and the lamina dura.

## Detection of Extra Roots and Canals

As was seen in Chapter 3 abnormalities in the root anatomy can occur in any tooth. Generally if the anatomy deviates from the normal the root canal system will also be likely to be abnormal. For this reason preoperative radiographs should be examined very carefully preferably with a magnifying glass. Any variation of the outline or contour of the root should make one suspect an extra root. Sharp differences in density of the radiographic picture of roots are often indicative of the presence of an extra root.

Extra canals cannot be distinguished easily on the preoperative X-ray and the diagnostic wire radiograph may be more useful. In such instances it is possible to follow the diagnostic reamer or file within the root canal and if an extra canal is present it will show as a dark line adjacent to the reamer. This line need not be parallel to the reamer but may be seen to leave the main canal, curve and rejoin further along the canal (Slowey, 1974).

The coronal third of the root should be examined carefully because the root canal is generally widest in this area. A sharp change in density along the canal may be due to a divergence of the main canal into two finer branches. Divergent canals often rejoin a short distance from the apical foramen and this can be demonstrated by placing a reamer to within 1 mm of the foramen and then attempting to negotiate the second canal to the same point. If the second reamer binds well short of the calculated length then it can be assumed safely that the canal joins at that point. Rubber dam clamps often obscure the coronal third of the root canal because the angulation of the tube throws a shadow onto the X-ray film.

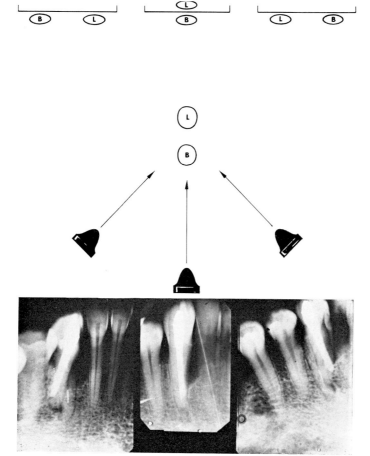

*Fig.* 98. Diagrammatic representation of three X-rays showing the principle of 'parallax shift'.

Certain teeth, e.g. the upper first premolars and the lower incisors, may have two canals in a buccolingual direction one behind the other. These canals are usually superimposed on the radiograph and it may be useful if such teeth are routinely X-rayed from different angles. In this way the extra canal can be demonstrated and it is also possible to determine the buccolingual position of each root. As can be seen from *Fig.* 98 the median angle picture shows the superimposed canals. If the tube is now moved 20° in either direction and a further X-ray taken the root nearest the tube appears to move, relative to the other root, in the opposite direction to the tube movement. This technique is known as 'parallax shift'.

Radiographs must be as clear and undistorted as possible and this is generally possible in all quadrants of the mouth except the upper posterior. In these areas the use of a long cone technique enhances the quality of the radiograph because the longer the distance between the target of the X-ray apparatus and the object to be X-rayed the more parallel the X-ray beam. This results in a diminished penumbra effect and less magnification and distortion. Often, long cone techniques are criticized because the exposure has to be increased proportionally. However, this does not result in an increased dose to the patient because he too is further away from the X-ray source (Smith, 1973).

## IV. OBSTRUCTIONS IN THE ROOT CANAL

Mention has already been made of the importance of studying carefully the preoperative radiograph, *prior* to beginning endodontic therapy. From the radiograph one should discover the course, length and approximate diameter of the root canal and also whether any obstructions will prevent instrumentation to the correct level. This information will determine the treatment plan for that particular tooth.

Whether it is necessary or possible to remove the obstruction will depend on its composition, size and position within the pulp cavity. Obstructions can be naturally occurring or iatrogenic.

### Natural Obstructions

Natural obstructions include pulp stones, calcified canals or anatomical anomalies which makes instrumentation impossible.

Provided *pulp stones* are identified from the X-ray and occur within the pulp chamber they present little difficulty in removal. However, it is more difficult to remove a stone from a root canal particularly if it is attached to the walls of the canal. In such instances one can only hope that the blockage is not complete and that a file can be passed alongside the stone which is removed by slow and careful filing.

*Calcified Canals*

Canals that are fully calcified from the pulp chamber to the apical foramen are very rare. Calcification normally begins in the pulp chamber and continues in an apical direction.

Sometimes canals that look completely calcified can be instrumented because there remains a very fine pathway within the calcified material. This is not visible on X-ray because the contrast on the film is inadequate. For this reason an attempt should always be made to find this fine pathway and the instrument of choice is No. 08 file used with a filing action only. Once this file has reached the correct level enlargement of the canal is a simple matter. The use of ethyline diamine tetra-acetic acid (EDTA) will often help this stage of the operation.

It must be made quite clear that a symtomless tooth with a calcified canal requires no treatment for it is possible that not only is the canal calcified, but also that the apical foramen has been occluded by the deposition of secondary cementum. Such a tooth should be kept under yearly X-ray review and if an area should develop the tooth can be treated surgically.

## Iatrogenic Obstructions

Iatrogenic obstructions include broken root canal instruments, posts, gutta percha or solid cement root fillings.

*Metallic Visible Objects*

If the fractured object is metallic and visible its recovery is relatively simple by using the Masserann technique described on p. 83.

*Invisible Metallic Fragments*

If the fragment is not visible its recovery becomes more difficult. Instruments broken close to the apex may, on occasions, serve as a satisfactory sectional root filling and may be accepted if the tooth remains symptomless. However, the patient should be told of the accident and yearly radiographic checks arranged.

If the fragment is causing symptoms and has to be removed then the following alternatives are possible and these will depend on the position, size and type of instrument broken.

If the instrument is fine and not jammed firmly within the canal then it may be possible to remove it by passing barbed broaches or Hedstroem files alongside it, entwining these around it, and lifting the fragment out of the canal.

If the fragment is larger then a channel has to be cut around it, and again the Masserann technique is sometimes useful.

Carbon steel instruments can often be made to rust by sealing in a freshly prepared solution of iodine in potassium iodide. This may require several applications over many visits. Sometimes it is not possible to remove a broken fragment from a canal because the risks of perforation are too great or because the removal entails the destruction of so much tooth substance that the remaining root and/or crown are too weak to support an adequate restoration. In such cases consideration should be given to surgical techniques and apicectomy, hemisection or elective replantation may have to be employed (see Chapter 8).

## Non-metallic Root Fillings

Single cone gutta percha root fillings are generally easy to remove by passing a coarse barbed broach, rat-tailed or Hedstroem file alongside the point and pulling the point in an incisal or occlusal direction. Removal becomes more difficult where a lateral condensation technique has been used. In such cases it may be necessary to soften the gutta percha with chloroform or xylol, but as these solvents act on a small portion of the gutta percha at a time root filling removal becomes much slower and more tedious.

The removal may be accelerated by using a Gates drill (see p. 72) and drilling out the bulk of the material. This operation should be carried out carefully lest the root be perforated.

Certain cement type root fillings that set hard may defy instrumentation and even direct drilling may not be possible. The hardness of the filling material and of tooth substance are so alike that tactile sense is lost and perforation occurs.

## Prevention

Generally instruments break because of abuse and, when such an accident occurs, it is difficult to justify it to oneself let alone to the patient.

Instruments break because they have been used too many times, have been over heated during sterilization or have been twisted excessively within the root canal.

Fine reamers and files (08–25) should only be used once and then discarded. Larger sizes may be sterilized and used again provided they are examined carefully and discarded if the blades show any irregularity, this being an indication of overuse.

The breaking of an instrument in a root canal is distressing to the patient and its retrieval very time consuming. For these reasons the use of imperfect instruments is a false economy.

## V. IMMEDIATE ROOT THERAPY

The question is often asked whether a symptomless tooth, be it vital or non-vital, should be instrumented and root filled at the same visit. In the case of vital teeth it is argued that the canal is sterile and if the root filling is completed quickly the chances of infecting the canal are minimized. This is, of course, true but one must remember that inflammation may occur not only because of infection but also because of mechanical trauma.

The extirpation of a vital pulp is a traumatic incident and the blood vessels and nerve fibres are literally torn apart and this results in haemorrhage. If the blood vessels are torn within the root canal it is feasible that the haemorrhage can be arrested before the root filling is completed, or alternatively, during the obturation of the canal when a well condensed root filling will act as a pressure pack and prevent further haemorrhage. In such cases the patient will generally experience no after-pain.

However, if the severing of the blood vessels occurs periapically the haemorrhage will be into the periapical tissues and this will result in an inflammatory response, possibly with exudate formation. If the canal is sealed there will be no empty space into which the exudate can discharge and it is very likely that the patient will experience after-pain for two or three days. Protagonists of the immediate root filling suggest that analgesics and antibiotics should be prescribed as a routine to overcome this problem. This normally alleviates the symptoms but one questions the unnecessary prescription of these drugs.

Generally, it is safer if vital teeth are root filled in two visits. At the first visit the pulp is extirpated, the canal is prepared fully and the tooth dressed and sealed. This allows any periapical exudate to discharge into the empty canal which reduces considerably the chances of after-pain.

This argument is not valid in the case of symptomless non-vital teeth but even here it is safer if the root filling is carried out in two visits. In teeth where the canals have not previously been instrumented and medicated there is no guarantee that they are sterile. If they are not, infected material may be forced periapically and this may lead to complications as discussed above.

The only occasion when an immediate root filling may be safely carried out is when a tooth has been previously root filled and the root filling has to be partly removed in order to accommodate a post-retained restoration. In such instances the partial removal of the root filling generally leads to disturbance of the apical seal as well (Neagley, 1969) and it may be safer to remove it entirely and replace it with a sectional root filling before proceeding to the construction of the post crown.

217

## VI. THE ENDODONTIC TREATMENT OF FRACTURED TEETH

The treatment will depend on the site and type of fracture which can be simple or comminuted, single or multiple, horizontal or vertical, coronal or radicular.

A simple classification might be—

1. *Crown fractures* involving
   *a.* Enamel only
   *b.* Enamel and dentine without pulp exposure
   *c.* Enamel and dentine with pulp involvement.
2. *Root Fractures*
   *a.* Vertical
   *b.* Horizontal
      i. In the cervical third
      ii. In the mid-third
      iii. In the apical third.

### 1. *Crown Fractures*

The management of crown fractures has been discussed on p. 58.

### 2. *Root Fractures*

The endodontic treatment of teeth with root fractures should be considered together with the subsequent restorative treatment to the crown. There is no point in saving a root that cannot be subsequently restored.

*a. Vertical fractures* in single rooted teeth have a hopeless prognosis because it is not possible to either stabilize the fragments or remove one part surgically and leave the other in situ.

The prognosis of vertically fractured multi-rooted teeth will depend on the site of the fracture. Sometimes it is possible to hemisect the tooth and retain the strong root or roots which have to be root filled conventionally. (*See* pp. 161, 199.)

*b. Horizontal Fractures*

i. IN THE CERVICAL THIRD OF THE ROOT treatment will depend on whether the fracture line extends above or below the alveolar bone crest.

If above, the root canal should be filled with an apical fifth root filling and the gingival tissue above the fracture line removed surgically so that it is possible to obtain a satisfactory impression for a post-retained restoration.

Sometimes the two fragments remain in contact after fracture. In such cases it is often useful if an impression of the arch is taken prior to the extraction of the crown so that the crown can be replaced in the impression and a model fabricated. This model will

218

have an accurate reproduction of the fractured root surface and a temporary post crown can be constructed which will be accurate and lessen the irritation of the gingival tissues between the fracture line and the gingival margin. Alternatively the patient's fractured crown itself can be utilized as a temporary restoration until the gingival tissues have healed following the periodontal surgery.

If the fracture extends below the crest of the alveolar bone treatment becomes more difficult because it is impossible to construct a satisfactory, well fitting restoration.

The root filling is again a simple matter and should be of the sectional variety.

The conservative problem can be tackled in two ways. If the fracture is not too deep within the alveolar bone, the root face can be exposed by periodontal surgery and the removal of alveolar bone. The disadvantage of this technique is that it alters the gingival line which may make treatment aesthetically unacceptable to the patient.

A second technique has been suggested by Heithersay (1973) and consists of an endodontic, orthodontic and conservative approach. The tooth is root filled with a sectional root filling and a retentive post and core unit, preferably of a screw post type such as the Kurer anchor system*, is fixed in the canal. The root is then moved orthodontically in a vertical direction until the root face is in a position that will allow the taking of a satisfactory impression for crown restoration.

ii. IN THE MID THIRD OF THE ROOT: This type of fracture is probably the most difficult to manage because the removal of either fragment leaves insufficient tooth substance for successful long term restoration of the tooth. To overcome this problem the approach can be either conservative or surgical and in each case the aim is to preserve, or even improve the crown-to-root ratio.

*a. Conservative:* If the fracture is simple, the fragments in opposition and the pulp vital it may be worth while to attempt the conservative union of the fragments. The crown is freed from any occlusal load and immobilized by splinting to the adjacent teeth. This can take the form of wire and acrylic ligatures, acrylic or cast splints, cemented over the whole arch, orthodontic banding or wire and an acid etch technique which gives more aesthetically pleasing results.

Once the tooth is immobilized it is possible that a fibrous union will take place between the two fragments. Rarely the union may be by calcific repair tissue which, according to Manley and Marsland (1952), consists of both tubular dentine and uncalcified organic matrix.

---

*Kurer Anchor System: Cottrell & Co., 15–17 Charlotte St., London W1.

The splint should remain in position for 2 or 3 months and the tooth kept under observation indefinitely both by vitality tests and radiographically. Success will depend on the closeness of the root fragments, the efficiency of the immobilization and the lack of infection.

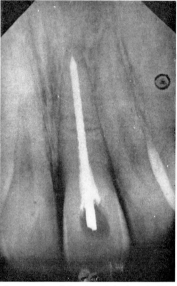

*Fig.* 99. Root fragments of fractured incisor held together with a Hedstroem file which also acts as the root filling point.

If the fragments are in close apposition but the pulp is non-vital or irreversibly injured then it is possible to splint the fragments through the root canal. As the root fragments are in close apposition one is able to prepare the root canal conventionally and root fill the tooth with a post that is strong enough to immobilize and hold both fragments together. This can take the form of a nickel-chrome post, or a Kerr 'Endopost' or a 'K' type or Hedstroem file (*Fig.* 99). In many ways a file is preferred for it can be 'screwed' and cemented in position, so that its retention is enhanced at least in the apical fragment. The coronal end of the file is severed, within the access cavity, with a turbine and stabilized with a well condensed amalgam filling.

*b. Surgical:* The above conservative techniques are not possible if the fracture is comminuted or if the fragments are not in reasonably close apposition. In such cases the approach must be surgical and can take the form of apicectomy, removal of the apical fragment or fragments and retrograde root filling. This is only possible if it is considered that the remaining root fragment will be adequate to support the crown.

If it is not, then an endodontic endosseous stabilizer offers the only other solution (*see* p. 166).

iii. IN THE APICAL THIRD OF THE ROOT: This is probably the easiest type of fracture to manage and can be by the conservative techniques described above (iia) or by surgical treatment. In the latter case an apicectomy with retrograde or through-and-through filling is all that is necessary.

*Recall*

Mention has been made of the necessity of frequent and careful postoperative checks. These are particularly necessary in the conservative management of vital teeth and in those teeth that have been splinted through the root canal, because resorption of the fragments at the site of the fracture is not infrequent and when it occurs it progresses rapidly.

REFERENCES

Bender I. B. and Seltzer S. (1961) Roentgenographic and direct observation of experimental lesions in bone, I and II. *J. Am. Dent. Assoc.* **62,** 152, 708.

Heithersay G. S. (1973) Combined endodontic–orthodontic treatment of transverse root fractures in the region of the alveolar crest. *Oral Surg.* **36,** 404.

Hudson M. W. P. (1960) *Digest Report of the Meeting of the Society for the Advancement of Anaesthesia in Dentistry.* 1 December 1960.

Jorgensen N. B. (1960) *Digest Report of the Meeting of the Society for the Advancement of Anaesthesia in Dentistry.* 1 December 1960.

McEwan T. E. (1974) Premedication, general anaesthesia and sedation in outpatient dentistry. In: Harty F. J. and Roberts D. H. (ed.), *Restorative Procedures for the Practising Dentist.* Bristol, Wright, p. 103.

Manley E. B. and Marsland E. A. (1952) Tissue response following tooth fracture. *Br. Dent. J.* **93,** 199.

Manson J. D. (1963) The lamina dura. *Oral Surg.* **16,** 432.

Neagley R. L. (1969) The effect of dowel preparation on the apical seal of endodontically treated teeth. *Oral Surg.* **28,** 739.

Regan J. E. and Mitchell D. F. (1963) Evaluation of periapical radiolucencies found in cadavers. *J. Am. Dent. Assoc.* **66,** 529.

Roberts D. H. and Sowray J. H. (1970) *Local Analgesia in Dentistry.* Bristol, Wright.

Slowey R. R. (1974) Radiographic aids in the detection of extra root canals. *Oral Surg.* **37,** 762.

Smith N. J. D. (1973) Radiography and radiology for the dental practitioner. I, The dental X-ray set. *Br. Dent. J.* **134,** 434.

Wengraf A. (1964) Radiologically occult bone cavities: An experimental study and review. *Br. Dent. J.* **117,** 532.

# INDEX